AF679022

This work: "Care in Healthcare: Reflections on Theory and Practice", was originally published by Palgrave Macmillan and is being sold pursuant to a Creative Commons license permitting commercial use. All rights not granted by the work's license are retained by the author or authors.

Cover Image Credit/Copyright Attribution: IIerlok_Xolms/Shutterstock

Franziska Krause • Joachim Boldt
Editors

Care in Healthcare

Reflections on Theory and Practice

Editors
Franziska Krause
University of Freiburg
Freiburg, Germany

Joachim Boldt
University of Freiburg
Freiburg, Germany

https://doi.org/10.1007/978-3-319-61291-1

© The Editor(s) (if applicable) and The Author(s) 2018. This book is an open access publication.
Open Access This book is licensed under the terms of the Creative Commons Attribution 4.0 International License (http://creativecommons.org/licenses/by/4.0/), which permits use, sharing, adaptation, distribution and reproduction in any medium or format, as long as you give appropriate credit to the original author(s) and the source, provide a link to the Creative Commons license and indicate if changes were made.
The images or other third party material in this book are included in the book's Creative Commons license, unless indicated otherwise in a credit line to the material. If material is not included in the book's Creative Commons license and your intended use is not permitted by statutory regulation or exceeds the permitted use, you will need to obtain permission directly from the copyright holder.
The use of general descriptive names, registered names, trademarks, service marks, etc. in this publication does not imply, even in the absence of a specific statement, that such names are exempt from the relevant protective laws and regulations and therefore free for general use.
The publisher, the authors and the editors are safe to assume that the advice and information in this book are believed to be true and accurate at the date of publication. Neither the publisher nor the authors or the editors give a warranty, express or implied, with respect to the material contained herein or for any errors or omissions that may have been made. The publisher remains neutral with regard to jurisdictional claims in published maps and institutional affiliations.

Acknowledgement

This book was devised on the basis of a summer school on care in healthcare held in Freiburg, Germany, in 2015. The editors of this volume who were also the organisers of this summer school wish to thank the German Federal Ministry of Education and Science (BMBF) for financing the event and this publication (grant no. 01GP1485). We are glad that all of the participants of the summer school were willing to contribute to this book. We would also like to thank the Head of our department, Giovanni Maio, to join the group of contributors; as well as Johanna Feuchtinger, nursing quality management at Freiburg University Hospital, Annemarie Mol, Professor of Anthropology at Amsterdam University; and Christof Veit, Head of the Institute for Quality and Transparency in Healthcare (IQTIG) in Berlin for presenting at the summer school and taking part in the group discussions. Last but not least, we would like to thank Jonas Christoph and Marlene Reincke for unifying bibliography and citation styles.

Freiburg, Germany
January 2017

Franziska Krause, Joachim Boldt

Contents

Understanding Care: Introductory Remarks 1
Franziska Krause and Joachim Boldt

Framing Care 11

Forgotten Approaches to Care: The Human Being as Neighbour in the German-Jewish Tradition of the Nineteenth Century 13
Elisabeth Conradi

Nursing as Accommodated Care: A Contribution to the Phenomenology of Care. Appeal, Concern, Volition, Practice 37
Björn Freter

Fundamentals of an Ethics of Care 51
Giovanni Maio

The Interdependence of Care and Autonomy 65
Joachim Boldt

Caring Relationships: Commercial Surrogacy and the Ethical Relevance of the Other 87
Franziska Krause

Situated Care 109

Sociomaterial Will-Work: Aligning Daily Wanting in Dutch Dementia Care 111
Annelieke Driessen

The Dementia Village: Between Community and Society 135
Tobias Haeusermann

Regulation as an Obstacle to Care? A Care-Ethical Evaluation of the Regulation on the Use of Seclusion Cells in Psychiatric Care in Flanders (Belgium) 169
Tim Opgenhaffen

Witnessing as an Embodied Practice in German Midwifery Care 191
Annekatrin Skeide

Tensions in Diabetes Care Practice: Ethical Challenges with a Focus on Nurses in a Home-Based Care Team 211
Pei-Yi Liu and Helen Kohlen

Caring About Care in the Hospital Arena and Nurses' Voices in Hospital Ethics Committees: Three Decades of Experiences 237
Helen Kohlen

Towards a Three-Dimensional Perspective of Space for Humanizing Hospital Care 265
Hanneke van der Meide

Conclusion: Asking the Right Questions 283
Joachim Boldt, Annelieke Driessen, Björn Freter, Tobias Haeusermann, Franziska Krause, Pei-Yi Liu, Tim Opgenhaffen, and Annekatrin Skeide

Index 293

List of Tables

Table 1 Tronto's four-phase model with the corresponding ethical elements of an ethics of care, modified according to Conradi (2001) 52

Understanding Care: Introductory Remarks

Franziska Krause and Joachim Boldt

"Care" is without doubt among the most important concepts in healthcare. The very word "healthcare" bears witness to this fact, indicating what the healthcare system as a whole and the individual actions taking place within healthcare are all about—namely, to provide care. The concept of care plays an important role for the professional identity of caregivers, and it is part of the expectation of care receivers. This can easily be forgotten given that in public and academic discourse, issues such as costs, prevention, the just distribution of scarce resources and the patient's personal responsibility often figure more prominently than care.

Care is not only a descriptive concept, it also conveys a normative orientation. The term "care" enables one to evaluate different courses of action in healthcare. What is more, different courses of action can correspond more or less closely to what one perceives as good care. As there are standards and guidelines for and best practices of good care, care providers can ask themselves whether what they do constitutes good care. The question of whether the healthcare system as a whole as well as specific

F. Krause (✉) • J. Boldt
Department of Medical Ethics and the History of Medicine, University of Freiburg, Freiburg, Germany

© The Author(s) 2018
F. Krause, J. Boldt (eds.), *Care in Healthcare*,
https://doi.org/10.1007/978-3-319-61291-1_1

regulations and practices within healthcare live up to the ideals of good care is always subject to debate.

For example, one may ask whether it is good care in midwifery to allow mothers to give birth at home and to offer them support in doing so. Many factors must be taken into account in order to come to a conclusion—from the percentage of home and hospital births that involve severe incidents, to the experiences of mothers giving birth in both situations, to the costs of these two alternatives. These factors are related to different norms and may point in different directions. In order to find ways to proceed, one has to weigh these norms, including the well-being of mother and child, the economic and societal sustainability of healthcare provisions, and parents' preferences.

Socioeconomic stability may interfere with good care in individual cases, since, for example, the amount of time care providers can allocate to individuals is limited by the number of cases they are expected to manage. Determining what constitutes good care is hence usually a matter of finding reasonable compromises. In healthcare settings, a typical compromise involves finding a balance between optimal care for individuals on the one hand and the institutional demands of providing care to many care receivers over long periods of time as well as the limits of what can legitimately be asked of individual care providers on the other.

Approaches to the ethics of care have shown that care can indeed be understood as an overarching normative concept that integrates different normative orientations. In the current literature, the unifying role of care has been stressed, first and foremost, with regard to personal, dyadic relations as well as with regard to justice and political theory more generally (Conradi 2001; Groenhout 2004; Held 2006; Pettersen 2008; Pulcini 2013; Sevenhuijsen 1996). These approaches can be applied to healthcare. For example, if there is a conflict between care for the well-being of an individual mother and her child and the just allocation of institutional resources, the latter orientation can be understood as an attempt to safeguard the conditions that enable professional care in individual cases. Although protecting the well-being of an individual mother and her child is a prime example of caring, securing institutional socioeconomic stability can be understood as serving the prior aim of caring as well, since the ability to provide professional care in individual cases presupposes institutional stability. Making use of care as an overarching normative concept can guide this process of determining the best compromises. Institutional demands that cannot be justified on the basis of maintaining the care institution's socioeconomic stability may be rejected if they interfere with good care in individual cases.

Defining Care

In order to understand care, one may start by attempting to devise a general definition of this term. Such a definition of care must necessarily be broad if it is to cover as many important aspects of the phenomenon as possible. Care in healthcare comprises many elements including the physical interactions between care providers and patients, the observation of hygiene requirements and the completion of paperwork. Joan Tronto and Bernice Fisher have offered an influential definition that classifies as care all activities that help to "maintain, continue and repair 'our' world so that we can live in it as well as possible" (Tronto 1993, p. 40).

This definition can be fruitfully adapted to the healthcare context by replacing the term "activity" with "action", which specifically indicates goal-directedness and intentionality. Healthcare activities are triggered by patient needs and requests; they follow professional obligations, and are shaped by institutional demands. Thus, activities in this field are usually goal-directed, which is to say they are actions rather than activities. In the same vein, the verbs "maintain, continue, repair" may be changed to "maintain, improve, restore". While the first list describes the relations between people and all manner of entities, the second is tailored to actions that are directed towards humans and human health. On this basis, care in healthcare can be defined as follows:

Care in healthcare is a set of relational actions that take place in an institutional context and aim to maintain, improve or restore well-being.[1]

This definition brings to the fore three main aspects and characteristics of care that are of specific relevance in the healthcare system:

Relationality Personal relations are at the heart of care in healthcare, where the paradigm of care is the relationship between a person who gives care and another who receives care. According to this paradigm, relationality is understood as the ongoing verbal and non-verbal communicative process between physically present caregivers and care receivers. This presupposes attitudes like attentiveness and responsivity, which can have a decisive impact on care situations. The way patients perceive and react to the prospect of an unpleasant procedure can change significantly if the caregiver approaches the patient in a caring manner. Nonetheless, relationality in healthcare can also be less communicative and personal. For instance, in the case of surgery, it may be limited to the physician's physical intervention into a patient's body. In other instances, such as in telemedicine, care may take place without physical closeness between the caregiver and care receiver. Sometimes the relationality of care might even be completely invisible to observers. For example, when a physician completes a patient's files, there is no visible direct relation to the patient, although the intentions of this action are clearly relational.

Institutionality Care in healthcare is care in an institutionalised and professionalised context. In contrast to care in a private context, care actions in a healthcare setting are often standardised and subject to assessment. This institutional setting can be the source of normative tensions. For example, institutional rules and regulations that are only indirectly connected to the well-being of patients, such as doing paperwork, must be implemented in the daily routines of caregivers even though this diminishes their ability to directly engage with patients. Along the same lines, the rules and regulations concerning bedside caregiving often need to be adjusted to the needs of individual patients and their situation. It is unreasonable to expect that care can be fully standardised, which is to say that to a certain degree, care regulation will always have to leave room for individual, context-sensitive decisions. These normative tensions notwithstanding, regulation and standardisation can in many cases be regarded as being part of providing care for patients, since they enable, for instance, the long-term stability of healthcare systems and the just allocation of healthcare resources.

Well-being Care in healthcare is directed at those who are ill and at those who are at risk of becoming ill. In some cases, caring for a patient may simply mean curing that person, that is restoring health. In many other cases, such as chronic diseases and situations at the end of life, caring involves maintaining and improving the well-being of the patient to the extent to which this is still possible. Maintaining well-being in these cases is rooted in ongoing relational processes between caregivers and care receivers. As part of these processes, the understanding of well-being must be continuously adjusted, allowing caregiving to proceed in accordance with the wishes of the care receiver. Thus in principle, respecting patient autonomy does not conflict with caring for the patient's well-being.

At the same time, lending an ear to the patient might turn her initial denial into a willingness to attempt a new therapy. Care, therefore, inevitably involves the possibility of indirectly influencing a patient's will. What is more, there are instances of care where the current will, for example, of a dementia patient does not correspond to his overall well-being or his former will. In such cases, care might involve practices that directly influence the patient's will. In this context, it can be difficult to draw clear distinctions between manipulative actions that transgress the boundaries of care and those actions that still fall within the limits of care.

Understanding Care

As the aforementioned aspects of care make clear, a number of tensions and ambivalences emerge within the notion of care. Although a general definition of the term care can provide a better impression of the range of actions that this term covers, it will not help identify and normatively categorise these tensions, nor find ways to deal with them. However, the fact that it is difficult to come up with a precise definition of care does not imply that it is impossible to point out prototypical examples of care practices or to delineate a spectrum of more or less typical instances of care activities (Mol et al. 2010). To invoke a linguistics textbook example, one can name prototypical examples of objects that fall under the term "bird" or "animal" and give less common examples, such as penguins and corals, respectively, even if precisely defining these terms proves impossible.

In order to gain a better understanding of the meaning of care in healthcare in this sense, definitions must be supplemented by descriptions and analyses of concrete care practices. Referring to the tensions mentioned above, questions emerge that can only be answered with reference to concrete cases. For example: Can one's actions still be understood as being part of an ongoing communicative process with the patient? When do daily institutional routines support adequate caregiving, and when do they hinder giving care? Are one's actions still in line with what the patient wants and needs? This book supplies both reflections on general characteristics and definitions of care, and case studies that point to and analyse tensions within the notion of care in different healthcare settings.

Framing Care

Part one of this book deals with traditions of care theory, philosophical and anthropological approaches to care, and care as an overarching normative concept. Conradi highlights similarities between the notions and intentions of today's care ethics and those of Jewish social reform movements of the late nineteenth and early twentieth centuries in Germany. With regard to philosophical approaches, the book focuses on hermeneutic and phenomenological theories. The characteristics of personal relations, their inherent normativity and interpretations of human interaction have always been at the centre of these theories. Freter, in his contribution, follows the phenomenological tradition and focuses on the notion of the "appeal" that a person in need unwittingly directs at a potential caregiver, using the story of the Good Samaritan as a paradigmatic example. Maio shows how care ethics can be connected to central themes of the hermeneutic tradition, as exemplified by Paul Ricoeur. Care is often assumed to be an antagonistic concept to respect for autonomy. Referring to Ricoeur's concept of the self, Boldt argues instead that an adequate understanding of care necessarily incorporates respect for autonomy and vice versa. Krause highlights relationality and responsibility as parts of care. She turns to the case of commercial surrogacy and shows how care ethics and Emmanuel Levinas' notion of the Other add important and often neglected aspects to the ethical evaluation of surrogacy.

Situated Care

The second part of the book focuses on care in different healthcare settings and analyses cases that do not initially seem to fit within the care paradigm. Typically, these situations pose a challenge to any kind of clear ethical solutions. For example, as Driessen discusses, caring for persons with dementia in residential care homes may comprise elements of "working on the will" of the care receiver in order to align what the resident wants with what the caregiver deems necessary for the person's well-being. Haeusermann also addresses dementia care, describing care practices in the first German dementia village and analysing ambivalences between regulation and freedom, and the constant oscillation between social inclusion and exclusion. On the basis of the current Flemish regulation on the use of seclusion cells in psychiatric institutions, Opgenhaffen suggests that while caregivers should not be overwhelmed or blinded by regulation, regulation should not prematurely impose a rational-objective mode on care. Instead, he spells out how seclusion regulation and care could fruitfully co-exist. Skeide describes witnessing as the relational and environmentally structured strategy of midwives in Germany and France. Being able to witness can be an integrating experience or have an alienating effect. In either case, Skeide establishes that clinical settings tend to delimit witnessing as a midwifery care practice. Pei-Yi Liu's chapter focuses on providing care in the actual homes of diabetes patients. In doing so, she traces the ethical dilemmas and challenges healthcare professionals face when dealing with a chronic illness in homecare settings. She shows that nurses' care tasks alternate between notions of patient autonomy and professional authority—two concepts that at times seem unbridgeable. Kohlen contends that the specific care knowledge and care perspective of nurses is underrepresented in the clinical institutional communication, possibly resulting in harm for patients. On the basis of studies in nursing ethics, she examines the ethical problems faced by nurses providing hospital care and their participation in hospital ethics committees over the last 30 years. Van der Meide uses the conceptual tool of the "three dimensional space", introduced by the philosopher and sociologist Henri Lefebvre, in order to describe and delineate the humanising and dehumanising effects of care in the hospital. She shadowed older patients during their stay in the hospital. Their experience of the hospital environment leads to feelings of "not fitting in" and "not belonging to".

All of the contributions in this book highlight the role of care in healthcare. They cannot and do not intend to provide an exhaustive overview of the field. Nonetheless, we are convinced that they give valuable insights into core characteristics as well as tensions and ambivalences of the notion of care in healthcare.

Note

1. This definition has been discussed and developed jointly by many contributors of this book in the course of a workshop on care in healthcare held in Freiburg in September 2015 (Joachim Boldt, Annelieke Driessen, Björn Freter, Tobias Häusermann, Franziska Krause, Pei-Yi Liu, Tim Opgenhaffen, Annekatrin Skeide).

References

Conradi, E. (2001). *Take Care. Grundlagen einer Ethik der Achtsamkeit*. Frankfurt a.M.: Campus.

Groenhout, R. E. (2004). *Connected Lives. Human Nature and an Ethics of Care*. Lanham: Rowman & Littlefield.

Held, V. (2006). *The Ethics of Care. Personal, Political and Global*. Oxford: Oxford University Press.

Mol, A., Moser, I., & Pols, J. (2010). *Care in Practice. On Tinkering in Clinics, Homes and Farms*. Bielefeld: transcript.

Pettersen, T. (2008). *Comprehending Care*. Lanham: Lexington Books.

Pulcini, E. (2013). *Care of the World. Fear, Responsibility and Justice in the Global Age* (K. Whittle, Trans.). Dordrecht: Springer.

Sevenhuijsen, S. (1996). *Citizenship and the Ethics of Care. Feminist Considerations on Justice, Morality and Politics*. London: Routledge.

Tronto, J. C. (1993). *Moral Boundaries. A Political Argument for an Ethics of Care*. New York: Routledge.

Open Access This chapter is licensed under the terms of the Creative Commons Attribution 4.0 International License (http://creativecommons.org/licenses/by/4.0/), which permits use, sharing, adaptation, distribution and reproduction in any medium or format, as long as you give appropriate credit to the original author(s) and the source, provide a link to the Creative Commons license and indicate if changes were made.

The images or other third party material in this chapter are included in the chapter's Creative Commons license, unless indicated otherwise in a credit line to the material. If material is not included in the chapter's Creative Commons license and your intended use is not permitted by statutory regulation or exceeds the permitted use, you will need to obtain permission directly from the copyright holder.

Framing Care

Forgotten Approaches to Care: The Human Being as Neighbour in the German-Jewish Tradition of the Nineteenth Century

Elisabeth Conradi

Jewish Ethics in Germany

In the United States and Europe, the ethics of care has achieved a prominent position among the variety of normative views in circulation.[1] A major exception is the German-speaking world, which has for the most part ignored the topic and the feminist perspectives that often accompany it.[2] Indeed, the entire subject area—along with the related concepts of benevolence, attention, donation, hospitality, and empathy—has hardly played a role in German university philosophy over the centuries, up to and including the present day. How to explain the German-speaking world's neglect? I would like to argue that philosophers advocating Jewish ethics in the nineteenth and early twentieth centuries planted the seeds

I would like to express my high regard to Dominic Bonfiglio for his competent and careful language revision from earlier drafts of this text into its final version.

E. Conradi (✉)
Baden-Wuerttemberg Cooperative State University (DHBW),
Stuttgart, Germany

© The Author(s) 2018
F. Krause, J. Boldt (eds.), *Care in Healthcare*,
https://doi.org/10.1007/978-3-319-61291-1_2

for these ideas but that their work was repressed by the Nazi regime and obscured by its long shadow, preventing a modern reception.

In 1935, Martin Buber (1878–1965) published *Der Nächste*, a collection of four essays on what it means to relate to other human beings as neighbours by the Marburg philosopher and neo-Kantian Hermann Cohen (1842–1918). In the introduction, Buber discusses when and under what circumstances assistance should be provided to others (1935, p. 7). He defends the need for positive duties against the widely held view in philosophy that restricts ethical duties to the ancient dictum 'Do no harm'. This position generally holds action to be mandatory only in very exceptional cases (Conradi 2016, pp. 54–58). Even a philosopher like Arthur Schopenhauer, who saw compassion as the driving force behind ethical behaviour, believed that the need must be acute and the emergency dire before action is required (2005, p. 101). For contemporary philosophers following Schopenhauer's lead, the main criteria for performing individual assistance are an expectation of a significant effect, a severe emergency, a limited duration of aid, and a minor effort required for assistance (Mieth 2012, p. 243). Buber focuses on two other aspects of positive duty: whether the recipient is a member of one's own collective and whether the recipient is spatially proximate. Buber emphasises that the person at the receiving end could be anyone and therefore no distinction should be made between neighbour, stranger, friend, acquaintance, and enemy. But he believes particular attention should be paid to any person who is within the helper's immediate sphere:

> 'Be loving to your fellow as to one who is like you', is written in the Scripture, and shortly thereafter, as if to avoid any misunderstanding at any time, through special highlighting: 'Be loving to a stranger as to one who is like you'. Rea, the fellow, is someone I am dealing with, whom I met just now, the human being so to speak, for whom I should be 'concerned' at this moment, whether he is of my own people or a foreigner. I should, literally translated, 'love *him*': turn towards him tenderly, show him love, practice love; namely as someone who is 'like me': in need of love such as I, in need of an act of love of a rea like me—as I know it just from my own soul. That this is to be understood in this way arises from the words following the second sentence: 'Because you've been strangers in the land of Egypt'—or, as it says more clearly elsewhere: 'You know the soul of the stranger,

> because you've been strangers in the land of Egypt'. You know this soul and its suffering, you know what it needs, and therefore, those to whom it was once refused, deny them not! Let us dare, from there, to put the justification of the first sentence in words. Be loving to your fellow human being as to one who is like you—you know the soul of the co-human [*Mitmensch*], who is in need, so that one is loving to him, because you are people and you suffer yourself the plight of man. Such is a message of the 'Old Testament' (1935, pp. 6–7).

Buber stresses the equal ranking of human beings in one's proximity. For all of them, the same personal support is mandatory, regardless of whether they are neighbours, mere acquaintances, or strangers. Buber makes the impression that the act of assistance is less important than the act of turning our attention towards others. What ethical behaviour is truly about is the decency, attention, warmth, and kind-heartedness that accompany it. We should view others as in "need of love" [*liebesbedürftig*], we should "turn towards them tenderly" [*liebend zuwenden*], "show them love" [*Liebe erzeigen*], and "practice love to them" [*Liebe antun*] (1935, p. 6).[3]

Martin Buber was by no means alone in his focus on what it means to relate to other human beings as neighbours. In the long nineteenth century, religious philosophers, writers, and rabbinic scholars widely reflected on social justice, companionship, consolation, and cooperation. Around 30 texts written between 1837 and 1913 on this subject matter were recently republished under the title *Nächstenliebe und Barmherzigkeit* (Brocke and Paul 2015). Few of these texts were likely to have been written as contributions to contemporary philosophical debate. Many came in response to vehement attacks against the authors, with some critics even questioning their right to citizenship and societal belonging. What is more, the authors of these texts geared them towards lay readers in an effort to expand their knowledge and perhaps to equip them with arguments against common criticisms. The majority of these treatises were dedicated to defending Jewish ethical teachings against popular misrepresentation. They explicitly rebutted legends and obvious simplifications—such as the claim that the code of conduct Jews followed among themselves was different from the one they followed among non-Jews—and rejected the mischaracterisation of Jewish ethical teachings as small minded and petty. Jobst Paul argues that Jewish ethics ties the institutional social justice with individual ethical requirements of benevolence and charity (Paul 2015, p. 12). "In view of the complexity and depth with which these themes are meaningful for and mould Judaism in its ethical core", he observes, "it is completely incomprehensible that precisely this ethical core … became the ideological basis for hostility towards Jews" (2015, p. 13). But that is exactly what happened in the course of the nineteenth century: the process through which the Jewish minority had become equal citizens before the law was discredited. Underlying the calls for the revocation of Jews' citizenship and the criticisms of Jewish ethics were two interlocking myths. The first, Paul explains, was that "in Judaism, only a *member of the brethren* is considered a fellow human being. … The Jewish view is supposed to be selfish and particular, that is, geared towards its own interests". The second was that "only Christianity has brought forth a universalist … altruistic ethics of neighbour love, making Judaism obsolete" (2015, pp. 13 f.).

Hermann Cohen, in correcting such "misunderstandings" (1935d, p. 19), sought to elucidate the idea of *Mitmenschlichkeit*, or co-humanity, in the Jewish tradition (Sieg 1997, p. 252). In 1888, the Royal District Court of Marburg asked Cohen to provide an expert opinion on the following proposal: "The law of Moses is only valid from a Jew to another Jew; it has no bearing on Goyim, whom you may rob and cheat" (Cohen 1888, p. 3). Hermann Cohen presented his answer in an essay titled "Neighbour Love in the Talmud" ("Die Nächstenliebe im Talmud") (1888, p. 1).

This paper was one of the four texts collected in Buber's *Der Nächste.*[4] The editor's afterword (it is unclear whether it was written by Martin Buber or Margarete Susman[5]) contains a summary of the allegations critics directed against Jewish ethics in the late nineteenth century:

> The main accusation against Judaism was that it was spiritually and practically surpassed by … Christianity's unconditional neighbour love. Theologians and antisemites are in agreement on this point. Theologians like Rudolf Kittel and Franz Delitzsch concluded from it Christianity's morally superiority; antisemites concluded from it Judaism's inferiority. Vulgar antisemitism alleged and still maintains that Judaism's ethical principles applied only to Jews and urged immoral behaviour towards non-Jews. (Cohen 1935a, pp. 82 f.)

The afterword notes that Cohen's papers were directed against past arguments—the theologian Rudolf Kittel died in 1929—but in deciding to republish four of Cohen's texts in 1935, Buber was addressing his own contemporaries. The Protestant theologian Gerhard Kittel (1888–1948)[6] published a brochure in 1933 titled "The Jewish Question" ("Die Judenfrage"), in which he invited Christians to endorse a piece of legislation enacted by National Socialists that permitted government authorities to fire Jewish professors, judges and other public servants at short notice (Kittel 1933).[7] Kittel asked whether such a radical legislation was still justifiable from an ethical, Christian standpoint (1933, p. 7).[8] His answer—the question was merely rhetorical—is clear: "We have established the unconditional demand that the struggle against Judaism must be led on the basis of an international and clear Christianity" (1933, p. 8).[9] Kittel expressly denied "the equal social ranking of Jews and their basis civil rights" (1933, p. 20) and unambiguously legitimises the revocation of their citizenship by assigning them the status of "guest" ("Gast") and "stranger" ("Fremdling") (1933, p. 46).[10] In lending credence to his point, Kittel observed that over 3000 years ago Jews had lived as strangers in Egypt, and hence should continue to do so today. Grotesquely, Kittel tried to justify his position by quoting Mosaic law: "'You shall give the poor his wages on the same day, before the sun sets: whether he belongs to your people, or *whether he's a stranger who lives in your country and behind your gates*' (5. Mos. 24,14; 27,19)" (1933, p. 57).[11]

Martin Buber immediately replied to these arguments (particularly the fallacious interpretation of the stranger's status in Mosaic law) in his 1933 "Open Letter to Gerhard Kittel", which appeared in the journal *Theologische Blätter* (Buber 2011). In the second edition of his brochure Kittel published a response to Buber, where despite the usual academic modus operandi he elected not to publish Buber's text alongside his own (1934, pp. 87–100). Buber's 1935 collection of essays by Cohen can be understood as a rejection of Kittel's absurd arguments. In fact, Gerhard Kittel did not think up his positions entirely on his own. Other theologians had already paved the way. For example, Adolf Stoecker (1835–1909) published a collection of speeches where he notes that "modern Judaism seems to pose a major threat to German national life" (Stoecker 1880, p. 5). In 1880, Stoecker signed an "antisemite petition" submitted to the

Prussian Prime Minister Otto von Bismarck. Its purpose was to undo the legal emancipation of the Jews of 1869, and demanded that the German nation rid itself of Jews' domination, limit their immigration, and exclude them from official posts (Conradi 2014, p. 231; Krieger 2003). Cohen rebutted arguments like these—specifically addressing those presented by the historian Heinrich von Treitschke [1879, p. 574]—in his 1880 "A Statement on the Jewish Question" (Cohen 2014). A few years later, Cohen published his expert opinion for the Royal District Court of Marburg, in which he discussed the treatment of strangers in the Jewish ethical tradition (Cohen 1888).

Helping Those Nearby

Philosophers tend to think that individuals are not obliged to help others if the need is small, if the expected effect of the aid only results in an improvement, if the assistance is continuous, or if the assistance is too taxing. Sometimes they allow the possibility of obligation if there is some kind of proximity to those in need. Onora O'Neill argues that some people are obliged to help others when they are *socially* close to them. Parents have 'special' (in contrast to 'universal') obligations towards their children: they are "held by some" and are merely "owed to specified others" (O'Neill 1996, p. 198). But the fulfilment of 'special' obligations is at the discretion of the individual, who decides who feels socially close, and whether and to what extent to fulfil them (O'Neill 1996, p. 251). Accordingly, this position leaves many questions open. One important question is, Whom to help?

For Hermann Cohen, the idea of co-humanity [*Mitmenschlichkeit*] suggests that the person receiving aid must be a fellow human being—*Nächster*, someone near. But is a neighbour someone who is spatially near or socially near? Cohen's concept of the "human being as a neighbour" ("vom Menschen als dem Nächsten") gives no indication of pre-existing social proximity. Cohen does link co-humanity to a certain spatial closeness, however, and this is how Buber interprets Cohen's co-humanity (1935, pp. 6–7). For Buber, the neighbour is someone "with whom I have contact, whom I am just now meeting, the human being who concerns me at this moment" (1935, p. 6). Cohen talks about how the concept of the human being as neighbour and fellow human comes to be and reinterprets the "love of strangers" as a "creative moment" in this development (1888, p. 8). In this respect, there is no doubt for Cohen that the benevolence that accompanies co-humanity is directed at strangers and acquaintances in equal measure (Hollander 2012, p. 106). Whether someone counts as a 'co-human' [*Mitmensch*] depends only on whether the person is in difficulty and currently within one's own sphere. "Neighbour love, benevolence towards *the stranger as defined by nationality and religion*", he concludes, "is a commandment of Judaism" (1888, p. 8).

> In addition to stranger love, Cohen stresses the basic requirement of social equality of human beings and their 'co-humans'. This kind of equality signifies parity and respect. In response to a comment by Naphtali Herz Wessely on the Third Book of Moses,[12] Cohen writes: "He doesn't say I should love the neighbour like myself but renders it as love thy neighbour, he is like you. This is the new idea: that people are equal to each other as human beings, namely as children made in the image of God. From this stems the possibility of the duty of neighbourly love. The duty does not stipulate the degree of love—which would raise the suspicion that neighbourly love was self-help. It teaches the equality of people and from this, love is derived" (1935b, pp. 17 f.).

As I observed above, Buber does not explicitly characterise neighbourly love as a feeling, but he does speak of love. By contrast, Hermann Cohen explains the relationship of the human being and the co-human by way of disposition [*Gesinnung*], which he believes leads to action. This disposition is not felt; actions unfold [*entfalten*] from it. After some time, an awareness [*Bewußtsein*] arises that connects people and expresses itself as solidarity:

> Neighbour love is a behaviour induced by a disposition towards co-humans, not the caution, protection, and defence against harm expected from them. All cultivation of a social life entails the unfolding of an ethical disposition. And compassion [*Mitleid*], which awakens people's suffering [*Leiden*], is less pain and passion than the dawning of moral awareness on behalf of the alliance of people, as a kind of force of nature that connects them. The disposition does not remain as an individual secret; rather, it expresses and is involved in the association of people (1935c, p. 8).

From the first sentence of this long passage, it is clear that Cohen understands the active support of others as a positive duty, not a negative duty limited to the omission of harmful acts. Cohen's sense of ethics goes beyond the individual; it encompasses the awareness that people are connected and gives reasons for solidarity among them.

Leo Baeck is another thinker who considers social equality to be a fundamental ethical idea. Like Cohen, Baeck does not believe that compassion is a feeling: "In complete fidelity to the sense and the actual content of the word, he says: 'Love your neighbour, he is like you'. The whole emphasis is located on this 'like you'. It expresses the unity of all that is human, a unity that makes life on Earth meaningful and which means much more than the indefinite word love. The *social idea* of one humankind and one human right and not merely a fleeting feeling has formed this idea" (2007, p. 11 f.). For Leo Baeck, to treat your fellow human being decently and kind-heartedly is not a question of feeling or individual decision. It is required of the individual and structures social life and interaction.

The German rabbi and writer Ludwig Philippson also argues against describing co-humanity as a feeling. He sees the commandment of neighbour love as a social duty to take action. In *Die That* ("The deed") Philippson writes, "Religion has not just brought God closer to people; it has also brought people close to the fellow human being" (1845, p. 250). Philippson distinguishes between two types of ethics. He claims the biblical injunction "Thou shalt love thy neighbour as thyself" for Judaism and reads it as the active support of fellow human beings. The other type of ethics appropriated the concept of neighbour love, mimicked it, and "embellished it with many other words, with lots of beautiful words, with many lovely sayings; people revelled in the feelings of love, of peace—but where was the deed?" (1845, p. 250). Placing the biblical quote in the context of rabbinic writings, Philippson contrasts this second type of ethics with Jewish assistance of others [*Wohltätigkeit*], which he describes as "the most beautiful, the most noble side of neighbourly love, wherein the word has fully become deed" (1845, p. 250). Philippson sees two branches of Jewish *Wohltätigkeit. Tzedaka*, which is often translated as "charity", refers to the aid we give those in need (1845, p. 250). It is mainly a question of financial support and donations in five cases: (1) freeing innocent prisoners; (2) funding weddings that people otherwise could not afford; (3) feeding and educating orphans; (4) providing food and lodging for travellers who have been displaced, are sick, or have an urgent reason to leave their homes; and (5) treating the poor with a kind heart and comforting words (1845, p. 251). The second branch of *Wohltätigkeit* is the *gemilut chassadim*. It consists (1) in the participation in wedding celebrations; (2) in prayer for and visit of the sick; in (3) unpaid volunteer cleaning, clothing and burial of the dead; and (4) in the "consolation of the bereaved and grieving" (1845, p. 252).

Tzedaka and *gemilut chassadim* are key ideas in Jewish ethics. *Gemilut chassadim* can perhaps be considered as 'lending a helping hand' or as in person social engagement (Zeller 1997, p. 117). In the *Jewish Encyclopaedia* of 1928, the entry for *gemilut chessed* translates it as a "demonstration of love" and as an "active participation in the joys and sorrows of the fellow human being". But it also involves assisting others (Elbogen et al. 2008, p. 1007). Philippson explains that both *tzedaka* and *gemilut chassadim* are to be exercised according to the extent of one's own powers and abilities, yet no one is exempt: "And behold, this is the deed! This is deed and reality! This is not only a word and a sweet sensation, but a strong deed. The wise say that even the poor person who live on alms should sometimes give alms!" (1845, p. 252)

Gemilut chassadim is a central concept in understanding the notion of common humanity's place in Jewish ethics. In Samson Raphael Hirsch's (1808–1888) translation of the treatise *Chapters of the Fathers* [*pirkei avot*], a part of the Mishnah, it is said that "the world relies on three things: on the Torah, on worship, and on deeds of love". Hirsch's translation was published posthumously in 1895. In his comment on the passage, he writes:

> *Torah*: the knowledge of the divine truth and the divine will for our whole inner and outer self and world life; *avoda*: the duty of obedience to God in fulfilling His will with our whole inner and outer self and world life; *gemilut chassadim*: the selfless deeds of love for the salvation of fellow human beings. These three things make up and complete the human world and what it encompasses depending on size and type; where they are missing, and if they are missing, and to the extent that they are missing, there is a gap that cannot be replaced by anything, a part of being is missing. … Without *gemilut chassadim*, humans lack the first part of being similar to

> God, and instead of bearing a likeness to God in saving and blessing their contemporaries, their hearts are frozen in senseless selfishness and hardness, and mankind lacks the bond of brotherhood and love, where the joy of life and happiness will thrive. In studying the Torah, human beings do justice to themselves; in *avoda*, to God; in *gemilut chassadim*, to their co-humans (1994, pp. 6f.).[13]

There are other interpretations of this line from the same decade. Isaak S. Bamberger (1863–1934) translates *gemilut chassadim* as "Wohltätigkeit" (contributing to wellbeing) and not, like Hirsch, as "selbstlose Liebestätigkeit" (selfless action out of love). Below Bamberger explains his decision:

> *The world rests on three things*—the world in its entirety as well as each one was created for the purpose of performing these three things: *the Torah;* the study of the Torah for one's own spiritual perfection is a duty for a human being unto himself. *Divine worship*, first in the sacrificial service in the Tabernacle and in the holy Temple of Jerusalem, and since the destruction of the latter, in prayer. This brings with it obligations toward God. *And assisting others*, through personal bodily assistance (visiting the sick, funerals, consoling the bereaved, sharing the joy of bride and groom, making peace and the like) and support of the needy and poor, which is suited to the duties toward the fellow human being (1981, pp. 2f.).

The forms of personal assistance described here were no mere lip service. They were practiced by cooperative associations, known as *hevrot* in Hebrew (Auerbach 1969, p. 19).[14] These non-profit groups had been active in large numbers and identifiable in every form in Europe since the sixteenth century (Farine 1973, p. 17; pp. 19f.; Baader 2001, p. 17).

Benjamin H. Auerbach, who wrote about the *hevrot* operating in Halberstadt in the nineteenth century, interprets such associations in the context of Jewish ethics:

> It is a fact that the first characteristic sign of the presence of a *pious* Jewish community is the existence of associations in their midst; they secure within the community the three pillars on which, according to the words of the wise, the world rests: knowledge of the Torah, religious and human *personal* service, and giving alms (Torah, avoda, and gemilut chassadim);

> specifically in creating a special association for *each* branch of assisting others. These special associations can be more active within those three very large spheres of influence (1866, p. 128).

Auerbach points out that the encouragement of these tasks was not to be achieved primarily through financial contributions, but through collectively coordinated voluntary activity in person (Auerbach 1866, p. 128, n. 1). Auerbach names the groups active in Halberstadt around 1866. Members of one association visited the sick, supported them financially, and assisted the dying. There was a "bread distribution society", a "firewood distribution association" (Auerbach 1969, p. 28) that provided fuel to "the local Jewish poor during the four months of winter" (1866, pp. 128f.), and an association that supported transients and the "itinerant poor" during holidays (1866, p. 128, n. 1). There was a male "burial society" (1866, p. 226), founded in 1769 (Farine 1973, p. 30), that dealt "with the washing and cleaning of the dead, accompanies them to the cemetery, and prepares their tomb" (Auerbach 1866, p. 128). There was also a women's association whose members visited women and girls in need, read and discussed books with them, and performed funerals (1866, p. 129). Hirsch B. Auerbach (1901–1973) describes a Halberstadt women's association whose statutes go back to 1492. It seems that this association was devoted primarily to the task of reading, and possibly to making clothes for the dead and visiting the sick (1969, p. 21). A soup kitchen was added at the beginning of the twentieth century (Auerbach 1969, p. 22).

All these activities are in line with the Jewish belief that people have a fundamental ethical obligation to their co-humans. Both in the Palestinian and Babylonian Talmuds, these obligations are defined as the exercise of mercy, hospitality, supporting the poor, visiting the sick, making peace, providing comfort for the grieving, and arranging funerals for the dead (Steppe 1997, pp. 81f.). Visiting the sick [*bikkur cholim*] also comprises the supply of food, the cleaning of the sick's room, the entertainment and consolation of the sick, and praying for them (Auerbach 1969, p. 27; Steppe 1997, pp. 81f.). Comforting, consoling, assisting, and, if necessary, nursing the sick, whether they are members of one's own community or outsiders, are part of religious duty in Judasim. Associations such as the hospital visit society [*chevrat bikkur cholim*] existed precisely for this purpose (Lewy 2008).

Lina Morgenstern places these associations specifically in the context of the German women's movement. In her book charting the history of this movement, she also mentions numerous Jewish women's associations for learning and alleviating distress. Morgenstern was aware of 700 such entities (Lordick 2013, p. 11) dedicated to supporting the poor, the sick, new mothers, orphans, and needy children (Morgenstern 1893, p. 140 ff.). Some ten years later, Siddy Wronsky described the establishment of the Jewish Women's League: "Founded in 1904 in Berlin by Berta Pappenheim, on the occasion of the meeting of the International Women's congress, it seeks to merge Jewish women's associations in Germany (1928: 10 national and provincial associations, 32 local groups, 450 individual associations) with the aim of promoting cultural and social Jewish tasks for women and by women, each with an equal voice" (Wronsky 1929). For more than 30 years, the Jewish Women's League set itself cultural, social, and feminist objectives (Daemmig 2004). This alliance formed out of common beliefs shared by Jewish social reformers such as Lina Morgenstern, Bertha Pappenheim (Pappenheim 2015), Alice Salomon (Salomon 1901), Sidonie Werner, and Henriette Fürth. Despite the differences between them, they all wanted to combine the care of the elderly and sick with the creation of vocational training institutions and merge child welfare with their educational ideas. Clearly, their social commitment in this regard went far beyond any of the positive obligations defended by philosophers. Indeed, behind their political and scholarly pursuits was a belief in the need for Jewish social ethics.

Political Practice and Ethical Belief

Margarete Susman also stresses the idea of practical engagement in her essay "Revolution and Women" [*Die Revolution und die Frau*], published in December 1918 (1992). She wrote her essay in the aftermath of the First World War and the subsequent November Revolution. By this time, the major goal of the women's movement had been achieved: political suffrage for women was introduced on 12 November 1918. Susman criticises the passivity of most women towards the beginning of the war and urges them to become involved in the revolution. This put Margarete

Susman in the proximity of radical feminists such as Lida Gustava Heymann and Helene Stöcker, who saw the introduction of women's suffrage as an admission of the collapse of male-dominated politics. By contrast, the speakers of the 'Federation of German Women's Associations' [*Bund Deutscher Frauenvereine*] issued a declaration in November 1918 that sought to justify the necessity of the war.

Susman begins her essay by asking why so few women in Germany were interested in politics, and discounts disenfranchisement and their lack of a public voice as reasons. She notes that suffragettes in England fought for their lives and the Germans only made fun of them, just as they had once distanced themselves from the "manly women" of the French and Russian revolutions. Although they possessed a "voluntary nature" arising from "self-sacrifice, silent goodness, pure heroism" (Susman 1992, p. 117), they lacked "freedom" in the sense of having made a "vital decision for or against what was happening" (Susman 1992, p. 118). German women's lack of political engagement was owing to the view that politics were "alien to the female character" (Susman 1992, p. 119); entering the political fray was tantamount "to a corruption of the purely human" (Susman 1992, p. 121).

But Susman argues that women are capable of being political and, given the politics of the time, their involvement was more needed than ever before. She proposes a politically active concept of the human opposed to what she criticises as "German inwardness" [*deutsche Innerlichkeit*]. A "ruinous inheritance of the great and inventive German metaphysics in uninspired times" (1992, p. 119), "German inwardness" is a situation in which individuals have no specific tasks but are occupied with general ideas. "Luther's isolation of individual conscience" was disastrous because the majority of Germans, especially women, were completely content "to be pure in their own eyes, untainted by personal guilt" (Susman 1992, p. 121). But women, Susman argues, applied the wrong criteria: "Women demanded from themselves that their actions be personal and good, righteous, helpful, and full of love. Any responsibility with regard to large life events as a whole was remote; their purpose here was that of serving faith. But faith can be moral only as religious behaviour; i.e. faith may only take place where our minds are faced with something basically inaccessible, something ultimate that we cannot fathom.

For all other purposes, faith is weakness and guilt" (1992, p. 123). This situation was created because of inadequate education, and Susman pins the blame on Protestantism, as underlined by her reference to Luther. In contrast to such inwardness "of serving faith" ("des dienenden Glaubens"), she describes Jewish religiosity as one of action.

In recent years, efforts have been made in Germany to revive aspects of the themes discussed above—say, how Buber's principal of dialogue informs professional care (Schwerdt 1998, pp. 261–320) or the relationship between care of others and the writings of Levinas (Krause 2015, p. 248). Yet the question remains why topics such as assistance, hospitality, empathy, care, listening, and help were confined to the margins of German-language philosophy until well into the 1990s. One cause of this relative silence may be actions taken during the National Socialist regime: Martin Buber was forced to leave Germany; the Jewish Women's League was dissolved in 1938 (Daemmig 2004); books were removed from libraries and publicly burned; writings by rabbis (Brocke and Paul 2015) and Jewish social reformers were systematically withdrawn from circulation; propaganda was introduced aimed at undermining solidarity between majorities and minorities (Schmidbaur 2002, pp. 129f.). Consequently, the German-language thinkers who endorsed ideas of mercy, benevolence, hospitality, assistance, and help went mostly overlooked in the second half of the twentieth century (Conradi 2015b).

About 100 years after Hermann Cohen wrote about what it means to relate to co-humans as neighbours, the psychologist Carol Gilligan wrote an empirically based study that introduces the idea of care as a specific way of viewing the world (1988b, p. 8), a world in which people are related to each other through human connection (1982, p. 29). In this, Gilligan shares common ground with Herman Cohen, who believes that assisting others results from an awareness that is developed over time. She describes her 'care perspective' as 'thinking in relationships', seeing people as members in a network of relations "on whose continuation they all depend" (1982, p. 29–30). She interprets communication and care not so much as activities but as aspects of a viewpoint (Conradi 2015a). The emphasis on awareness, not feelings, distinguishes Gilligan significantly from Schopenhauer and probably also from Buber. Schopenhauer believes that awareness can prevent us only from committing harm; assistance itself is motivated by feeling (2005,

p. 89). For attention and concern to be activated, "the distress" must be "great and urgent" (2005, p. 101). By contrast, Gilligan believes that action is needed when people are neglected and lonely (1988a, p. xviii); distance and detachment "constitute grounds for moral concern" (1987, p. 20). Buber, for whom despair is something that those who offer help know from their own experience, would agree (1935, p. 7). 'Thinking in relationships' is what allows us to recognise and identify such need in others. This point of view enables people to respond to depersonalisation in others by activating, cultivating, or repairing existing networks of communication (1987, p. 32).

Gilligan's 'thinking in relationships' goes far beyond what had previously been defended by the majority of philosophers as an ethical minimum: we must not only refrain from doing harm; we must improve others' situations. In this, she shares much with nineteenth- and early twentieth-century Jewish philosophy. Gilligan seems to agree with Buber that ethical commitment—whether conceptual or practical—applies first to those who are currently in one's own sphere. Yet she also agrees with Cohen that aid must *not* be limited to one's own social community; it ought to be extended to strangers as well. For Gilligan, social proximity between persons is constituted by 'thinking in relationships' through a type of anticipation; and it is established first and foremost through communicative engagement.

The ethics of care begins with human interactions—in assisting others effectively and in responding to human vulnerability and dependence. It starts off with everyday situations in which people assist others who require care for the foreseeable future, though their situation is not life-threatening. The ethics of care regards care-receivers as partners as well as co-subjects by emphasising interactions *between* human beings.

Notes

1. The discipline in which the ethics of care is discussed depends on country and language: in the Netherlands it is an object of study mostly in nursing science, gender studies, medicine, and theology (Vosman 2016); in the United Kingdom and in Sweden, it mainly appears in the social sciences; in France and Italy, it has been consigned to philosophy.

2. Even if the majority of German-speaking philosophers did not absorb the ethics of care I would like to highlight the work that had nevertheless been published. In Germany, there has been Andrea Maihofer's work on responsibility (Maihofer 1988) and Elisabeth Conradi's idea of attentiveness (Conradi 2001); in Austria, Christa Schnabl developed a socio-ethical theory of solicitude (Schnabl 2005, p. 439) and Herlinde Pauer-Studer has considered moral theory as it pertains to gender relations (Pauer-Studer and Nagl-Docekal 1993); in Switzerland, Annemarie Pieper has discussed the possibility of a feminist ethics (Pieper 1998) and Ina Prätorius has sketched out forms that a feminist ethics might take (Praetorius 1995). The care perspective has also appeared in debates about the increasing professionalisation in social work and nursing (Brückner 2008, 2010; Friese 2010; Schmid 2011). In the field of nursing, for example, Silvia Käppeli (2004) develops an idea of care from a theological point of view. In the area of social work, ethical approaches are occasionally taught that focus on the ethics of care (Großmaß 2006; Großmaß and Perko 2011, pp. 147–157; Noller 2007).
3. Buber leaves open whether he understands "love" as a deed, a feeling or an attitude.
4. Between 1894 and 1914 Cohen devoted three further essays to the question of what it means to relate to co-humans as neighbours.
5. The afterword is signed "M.S." but this might be a typo.
6. Gerhard Kittel was the son of Rudolf Kittel.
7. A significant number of the footnotes in the brochure cite Hitler's *Mein Kampf* and the political platform of the Nazi party ("Programm der NSDAP").
8. Kittel adds the following clarification: "For Christians, this truly brings up a serious question about the argument against the Old Testament and even the antisemitic attacks against the Jewish parts of the New Testament religion" (pp. 7 f). This passage, from the first edition of the brochure, was amended in the second edition (Kittel 1934): "For Christians, this truly brings up a serious question because for them, it is not only about humanity but about the problem of love, which is a fundamental requirement in Christianity and of which Paul the Apostle said that without it, everything else was nothing. On top of this, there is the multiple arguments of antisemites against the Old Testament; antisemitic attacks against the so-called Jewish components of the New Testament religion" (1934, p. 8).

9. In his brochure, Kittel, a professor of protestant theology, muses, "you can try to exterminate the Jews (pogroms)" ("man kann die Juden auszurotten versuchen (Progrome)") (p. 13), but proposes an alternative: "You can resolutely and consciously preserve the historical fact of a 'strangeness' between peoples" ("man kann entschlossen und bewußt die geschichtliche Gegebenheit einer Fremdlingschaft unter den Völkern wahren") (p. 13).
10. Kittel writes, "The right of the guest must be clearly demarcated against that of the citizen" ("das Recht des Gastes muß allerdings in aller Deutlichkeit gegen das des Bürgers abgegrenzt sein") (1933, pp. 39 f). And "*the status of the guest*" must be "restored" ("*entschlossen die Wiederherstellung des Gastzustandes* herbeizuführen") (1933, p. 38). "As soon as the principle of the right of strangers is absorbed into the (public) consciousness, it is absolutely clear and needs no further discussion that *a guest is not the holder of a public office, and cannot be a civil servant*" ("Sobald der Grundsatz des Fremdenrechtes ins Bewußtsein übergegangen ist, ist völlig klar und bedarf keinerlei weiterer Erörterung, *daß ein Gast nicht Inhaber eines öffentlichen Amtes, also nicht Beamter sein kann*") (1933, pp. 42 f.). Kittel mentions specific trades: "Once the idea of the guest is recognised and affirmed, it becomes obvious *that a stranger can be neither a teacher of German youth nor a professor*" ("Ist der Gedanke des Gastes einmal anerkannt und bejaht, so wird ferner selbstverständlich, *daß ein Fremdling im allgemeinen nicht Lehrer deutscher Jugend sein kann, auch nicht Hochschullehrer*") (1933, p. 46).
11. Kittel cites a similar passage in the same text. See Kittel 1933, p. 78, n. 21.
12. The comment of Naphtali Herz Wessely (1725–1805) was published in 1781. Moses Mendelssohn (1729–1786) translated the five books of Moses into German. Under the title *Sefer netivot ha schalom* ("The book of the ways of peace"), the translations (using Hebrew letters) were published between 1780 and 1783 by George Friedrich Starcke (Boeckler 2015, p. XIII). Mendelssohn and several others supplied commentary to the text.
13. Samson Raphael Hirsch's commentary was part of the book *Israel's Prayers* ("Sidur Tefilot Yisra'el"), which on nearly every page includes prayers in Hebrew, prayers in German, and commentary on the prayers in German (Hirsch 1895).

14. Hirsch Benjamin Auerbach (1901–1973) was a rabbi in Halberstadt from 1933 to 1938 and published on the history of the municipality. His great-grandfather Benjamin Hirsch Auerbach (1808–1872) was also a rabbi in Halberstadt, from 1863 to 1872, and, like his son, wrote about local history.

References

Auerbach, B. H. (1866). *Geschichte der israelitischen Gemeinde Halberstadt. Nebst einem Anhange ungedruckter, die Literatur, wie die religiösen und politischen Verhältnisse der Juden in Deutschland in den letzten zwei Jahrhunderten betreffender Briefe und Urkunden*. Halberstadt: Meyer.

Auerbach, H. B. (1969). Die Geschichte der alten Chewroth (wohltätigen Vereine) innerhalb der jüdischen Gemeinde in Halberstadt. *Zeitschrift für die Geschichte der Juden, 6*(1), 19–31.

Baader, B. M. (2001). Vom Rabbinischen Judentum zur bürgerlichen Verantwortung: Geschlechterorganisation und "Menschenliebe" im jüdischen Vereinswesen in Deutschland zwischen 1750 und 1870. In T. Adam & J. Retallack (Eds.), *Zwischen Markt und Staat. Stifter und Stiftungen im transatlantischem Vergleich* (pp. 14–29). Leipzig: Leipziger Universitätsverlag.

Baeck, L. (2007 [1918]). Die Schöpfung des Mitmenschen. In Verband der deutschen Juden (Ed.), *Soziale Ethik im Judentum* (pp. 9–15). Frankfurt am Main: Kauffmann.

Bamberger, I. S. (1981). Kommentar. In I. S. Bamberger (Ed.), *Pirke Aboth. Die Sprüche der Väter* (pp. 3–145). Basel: Goldschmidt.

Boeckler, A. M. (Ed.). (2015). *Die Tora nach der Übersetzung von Moses Mendelssohn*. London: JVFG.

Brocke, M., & Paul, J. (Eds.). (2015). *Nächstenliebe und Barmherzigkeit. Schriften zur jüdischen Sozialethik*. Köln: Böhlau.

Brückner, M. (2008). Kulturen des Sorgens über die Grenzen hinweg? *Polis, 49*, 9–28.

Brückner, M. (2010). Entwicklungen der Care-Debatte. Wurzeln und Begrifflichkeiten. In U. Apitzsch & M. Schmidbaur (Eds.), *Care und Migration. Die Ent-Sorgung menschlicher Reproduktionsarbeit entlang von Geschlechter- und Armutsgrenzen* (pp. 43–58). Opladen: Budrich.

Buber, M. (1935). Vorbemerkung. In H. Cohen (Ed.), *Der Nächste. Vier Abhandlungen über das Verhalten von Mensch zu Mensch nach der Lehre des Judentums* (pp. 6–7). Berlin: Schocken.

Buber, M. (2011 [1933]). "Offener Brief an Gerhard Kittel". In P. Mendes-Flohr (Ed.), *Martin Buber. Werkausgabe. Band 9. Schriften zum Christentum* (pp. 169–172). Gütersloh: Gütersloher Verlagshaus 2011.

Cohen, H. (1888). *Die Nächstenliebe im Talmud: Ein Gutachten dem Königlichen Landgerichte zu Marburg erstattet.* Marburg: Elwert.

Cohen, H. (1935a). *Der Nächste. Vier Abhandlungen über das Verhalten von Mensch zu Mensch nach der Lehre des Judentums.* Berlin: Schocken.

Cohen, H. (1935b[1894]). Über Wurzel und Ursprung des Gebots der Nächstenliebe. In H. Cohen (Ed.), *Der Nächste. Vier Abhandlungen über das Verhalten von Mensch zu Mensch nach der Lehre des Judentums* (pp. 11–18). Berlin: Schocken.

Cohen, H. (1935c[1910]). Gesinnung. In H. Cohen (Ed.), *Der Nächste. Vier Abhandlungen über das Verhalten von Mensch zu Mensch nach der Lehre des Judentums* (pp. 8–9). Berlin: Schocken.

Cohen, H. (1935d[1914]). Der Nächste. Eine kritische Untersuchung des biblischen Gebots der Nächstenliebe und seiner Mißdeutungen. In H. Cohen (Ed.), *Der Nächste. Vier Abhandlungen über das Verhalten von Mensch zu Mensch nach der Lehre des Judentums* (pp. 19–28). Berlin: Schocken.

Cohen, H. (2014 [1880]). *Ein Bekenntniß in der Judenfrage.* Berlin: Dümmler.

Conradi, E. (2001). *Take Care. Grundlagen einer Ethik der Achtsamkeit.* Frankfurt am Main: Campus.

Conradi, E. (2014). Eine Erörterung der "Antisemitenfrage" bei Constantin Brunner. In I. Aue-Ben-David, G. Lauer, & J. Stenzel (Eds.), *ConstantinBrunner im Kontext. Ein Intellektueller zwischen Kaiserreich und Exil* (pp. 230–253). München: De Gruyter.

Conradi, E. (2015a). Redoing Care: Societal Transformation Through Critical Practice. *Ethics & Social Welfare, 9*(2), 113–129.

Conradi, E. (2015b). Rekonstruierendes Quellenstudium und Nachrezeption: Wie die politische Ideengeschichte zu bereichern ist. In W. Reese-Schäfer & S. Salzborn (Eds.), *"Die Stimme des Intellekts ist leise". Klassiker/innen des politischen Denkens abseits des Mainstreams* (pp. 85–111). Baden-Baden: Nomos.

Conradi, E. (2016). Die Ethik der Achtsamkeit zwischen Philosophie und Gesellschaftstheorie. In E. Conradi & F. Vosman (Eds.), *Praxis der Achtsamkeit. Schlüsselbegriffe der Care-Ethik* (pp. 53–86). Frankfurt am Main: Campus.

Daemmig, L. (2004). Kampf um Gleichberechtigung: Der Jüdische Frauenbund. *HaGalil.com*. Retrieved December 5, 2016, from http://www.berlin-judentum.de/frauen/jfb.htm.

Elbogen, I. et al. (2008 [1928]). Gemilut Chessed. In G. Herlitz & B. Kirschner (Eds.), *Jüdisches Lexikon. Ein enzyklopädisches Handbuch des jüdischen Wissens in vier Bänden. Band II, D–H* (p. 1007). Berlin: Jüdischer Verlag.

Farine, A. (1973). Charity and Study Societies in Europe of the Sixteenth–Eighteenth Centuries. I. *Jewish Quarterly Review, 64*, 16–47.

Friese, M. (2010). Die ›Arbeit am Menschen‹. Bedarfe und Ansätze der Professionalisierung von Care Work. In V. Moser & I. Pinhard (Eds.), *Care - wer sorgt für wen?* (pp. 47–68). Opladen: Budrich.

Gilligan, C. (1982). *In a Different Voice: Psychological Theory and Women's Development*. Cambridge: Harvard University Press.

Gilligan, C. (1987). Moral Orientation and Moral Development. In E. Kittay & D. Meyers (Eds.), *Women and Moral Theory* (pp. 19–33). Totowa: Rowman and Littlefield.

Gilligan, C. (1988a). Prolog. In C. Gilligan, J. V. Ward, & J. M. Taylor (Eds.), *Mapping the Moral Domain* (pp. vii–xxxviii). Cambridge: Harvard University Press.

Gilligan, C. (1988b). Remapping the Moral Domain: New Images of Self in Relationship. In C. Gilligan, J. V. Ward, & J. M. Taylor (Eds.), *Mapping the Moral Domain* (pp. 3–19). Cambridge: Harvard University Press.

Großmaß, R. (2006). Die Bedeutung der Care-Ethik für die Soziale Arbeit. In S. Dungs, U. Gerber, H. Schmidt, & R. Zitt (Eds.), *Soziale Arbeit und Ethik im 21. Jahrhundert* (pp. 319–328). Leipzig: Evangelische Verlagsanstalt.

Großmaß, R., & Perko, G. (2011). *Ethik für soziale Berufe*. Paderborn: Schöningh.

Hirsch, S. R. (1895). Kommentar. In S. R. Hirsch (Ed.), *Israels Gebete (Sidur Tefilot Yisra'el)* (pp. 4–747). Frankfurt am Main: Kauffmann.

Hirsch, S. R. (1994 [1895]). Kommentar. In S. R. Hirsch (Ed.), *Pirke Avot. Sprüche der Väter* (pp. 1–123). Basel: Moraschа.

Hollander, D. (2012). Love-of-Neighbor and Ethics Out of Law in the Philosophy of Hermann Cohen. In C. Wiese & M. Urban (Eds.), *German-Jewish Thought Between Religion and Politics: Festschrift in Honor of Paul Mendes-Flohr on the Occasion of His Seventieth Birthday* (pp. 83–114). Berlin: De Gruyte.

Käppeli, S. (2004). *Vom Glaubenswerk zur Pflegewissenschaft. Geschichte des Mit-Leidens in der christlichen, jüdischen und freiberuflichen Krankenpflege*. Bern: Huber.

Kittel, G. (1933). *Die Judenfrage*. Stuttgart: Kohlhammer.

Kittel, G. (1934). *Die Judenfrage* (2nd ed.). Stuttgart: Kohlhammer.

Krause, F. (2015). Die Sorge des Menschen. In O. Müller & G. Maio (Eds.), *Orientierung am Menschen. Anthropologische Konzeptionen und normative Perspektiven* (pp. 241–255). Göttingen: Wallstein.

Krieger, K. (2003). *Der "Berliner Antisemitismusstreit" 1879–1881. Eine Kontroverse um die Zugehörigkeit der deutschen Juden zur Nation*. München: Saur.

Lewy, W. (2008 [1927]). Bikkur Cholim. In G. Herlitz & B. Kirschner (Eds.), *Jüdisches Lexikon. Ein enzyklopädisches Handbuch des jüdischen Wissens in vier Bänden. Band I, A–C* (p. 1038). Berlin: Jüdischer Verlag.

Lordick, H. (2013). Mildtätigkeit, Solidarität und Selbsthilfe – Jüdische und Wohltätigkeits- und Bildungsvereine im 19. Jahrhundert. In U. Stascheit & G. Stecklina (Eds.), *Jüdische Wohltätigkeits- und Bildungsvereine* (pp. 8–25). Frankfurt am Main: Fachhochschulverlag.

Maihofer, A. (1988). Ansätze zur Kritik des moralischen Universalismus. Zur moraltheoretischen Diskussion um Gilligans Thesen zu einer 'weiblichen' Moralauffassung. *Feministische Studien, 6*(1), 32–52.

Mieth, C. (2012). *Positive Pflichten. Über das Verhältnis von Hilfe und Gerechtigkeit in Bezug auf das Weltarmutsproblem*. Berlin: De Gruyter.

Morgenstern, L. (1893). *Geschichte der deutschen Frauenbewegung und Statistik der Frauenarbeit auf allen ihr zugänglichen Gebieten*. Berlin: Verlag der "Deutschen Hausfrauen-Zeitung".

Noller, A. (2007). Ethik der Achtsamkeit – Ethik der Menschenwürde: Sozialethische Anmerkungen zum Konzept Community Living. In T. Maas (Ed.), *Community Living. Bausteine für eine Bürgergesellschaft* (pp. 60–65). Hamburg: Alsterdorf.

O'Neill, O. (1996). *Towards Justice and Virtue: A Constructive Account of Reasoning*. Cambridge/New York: Cambridge University Press.

Pappenheim, B. (2015 [1899]). Frauenbewegung. In G. Wolfgruber (Ed.), *Bertha Pappenheim. Soziale Arbeit, Frauenbewegung, Religion* (pp. 92–97). Wien: Löcker. (Originally published under the pseudonym Paul Berthold).

Pauer-Studer, H., & Nagl-Docekal, H. (Eds.). (1993). *Jenseits der Geschlechtermoral. Beiträge zur feministischen Ethik*. Frankfurt am Main: Fischer.

Paul, J. (2015). Einleitung. In M. Brocke & J. Paul (Eds.), *Nächstenliebe und Barmherzigkeit. Schriften zur jüdischen Sozialethik* (pp. 7–19). Köln: Böhlau.

Philippson, L. (1845). Die That. In L. Philippson (Ed.), *Siloah. Eine Auswahl von Predigten. Zur Erbauung so wie insonders zum Vorlesen in Synagogen, die des Redners ermangeln* (pp. 245–253). Leipzig: Baumgärtner.

Pieper, A. (1998). *Gibt es eine feministische Ethik?* München: Fink.

Praetorius, I. (1995). *Skizzen zur feministischen Ethik.* Mainz: Matthias-Grünewald-Verlag.

Salomon, A. (1901). Die Arbeiterinnenbewegung. In H. Lange & G. Bäumer (Eds.), *Frauenbewegung und soziale Frauenthätigkeit in Deutschland nach Einzelgebieten. Handbuch der Frauenbewegung. Teil II* (pp. 205–216). Berlin: Moeser.

Schmid, T. (2011). Was heißt es in Zukunft, eine solidarische Gesellschaft zu sein? In ÖKSA (Ed.), *Langzeitpflege in einer solidarischen Gesellschaft - Herausforderungen und Chancen* (pp. 11–16). Wien: Info-Media.

Schmidbaur, M. (2002). *Vom 'Lazaruskreuz' zu 'Pflege Aktuell'. Professionalisierungsdiskurse in der deutschen Krankenpflege 1903–2000.* Königstein: Ulrike Helmer.

Schnabl, C. (2005). *Gerecht sorgen. Grundlagen einer sozialethischen Theorie der Fürsorge.* Freiburg im Breisgau: Herder.

Schopenhauer, A. (2005 [1840]). *The Basis of Morality* (A. B. Bullock, Trans.). Mineola: Dover.

Schwerdt, R. (1998). *Eine Ethik für die Altenpflege. Ein transdisziplinärer Versuch aus der Auseinandersetzung mit Peter Singer, Hans Jonas und Martin Buber.* Bern: Huber.

Sieg, U. (1997). Das Testament von Hermann und Martha Cohen. Stiftungen und Stipendien für jüdische Einrichtungen. *Journal for the History of Modern Theology, 4*, 251–264.

Steppe, H. (1997). *"... den Kranken zum Troste und dem Judenthum zur Ehre ...": Zur Geschichte der jüdischen Krankenpflege in Deutschland.* Frankfurt am Main: Mabuse.

Stoecker, A. (1880). Erste Rede. In A. Stoecker (Ed.), *Das moderne Judenthum in Deutschland, besonders in Berlin. Zwei Reden in der christlich-socialen Arbeiterpartei* (pp. 3–19). Berlin: Wiegandt und Grieben.

Susman, M. (1992 [1918]). Die Revolution und die Frau. In I. Nordmann (Ed.), *Das Nah- und Fernsein des Fremden. Essays und Briefe* (pp. 117–128). Frankfurt am Main: Jüdischer Verlag.

Treitschke, H. v. (1879). Unsere Aussichten. *Preußische Jahrbücher, 44*, 559–576.

Vosman, F. (2016). Kartographie einer Ethik der Achtsamkeit – Rezeption und Entwicklung in Europa. In E. Conradi & F. Vosman (Eds.), *Praxis der Achtsamkeit. Schlüsselbegriffe der Care-Ethik* (pp. 33–51). Frankfurt am Main: Campus.

Wronsky, S. (1929). Jüdischer Frauenbund. In G. Herlitz & B. Kirschner (Eds.), *Jüdisches Lexikon. Ein enzyklopädisches Handbuch des jüdischen Wissens in vier Bänden. Band III. lb–Ma* (p. 471). Berlin: Jüdischer Verlag.

Zeller, S. (1997). Soziale Arbeit und Judentum. Sozialethische Elemente professioneller Sozialarbeit/Sozialpädagogik. *Soziale Arbeit, 46*(4), 110–123.

Open Access This chapter is licensed under the terms of the Creative Commons Attribution 4.0 International License (http://creativecommons.org/licenses/by/4.0/), which permits use, sharing, adaptation, distribution and reproduction in any medium or format, as long as you give appropriate credit to the original author(s) and the source, provide a link to the Creative Commons license and indicate if changes were made.

The images or other third party material in this chapter are included in the chapter's Creative Commons license, unless indicated otherwise in a credit line to the material. If material is not included in the chapter's Creative Commons license and your intended use is not permitted by statutory regulation or exceeds the permitted use, you will need to obtain permission directly from the copyright holder.

Nursing as Accommodated Care: A Contribution to the Phenomenology of Care. Appeal, Concern, Volition, Practice

Björn Freter

Introduction

In this investigation, I will attempt to pinpoint the connection between nursing und care. On the one hand, I wish to understand the extent to which nursing represents a genuine normative practice, while on the other hand establishing how the normativity of this practice actually comes about. My hypothesis is as follows: nursing,[1] as I suspect and intend to investigate here, is to be understood as accommodated care.

It is not my intention to produce a normative draft determining what qualifies as caring or nursing and what does not. In order to verify the validity of this hypothesis, I first intend to develop a *phenomenology* of care.

I would like to thank Dinah Laubisch (Berlin), Kerry Jago (Bonn), Karoline Pietsch (Berlin), Annekatrin Skeide (Bremen) and Joachim Boldt (Freiburg) for helpful comments on first drafts of this text. I also wish to thank the Department of Neurology at the Schlosspark-Klinik (Berlin) for the opportunity to present and discuss a preliminary version of this work as part of an internal training workshop.

B. Freter (✉)
Independent Scholar, Berlin, Germany

© The Author(s) 2018
F. Krause, J. Boldt (eds.), *Care in Healthcare*,
https://doi.org/10.1007/978-3-319-61291-1_3

This phenomenological approach is, as far as I can tell, especially suited to an examination of caring and thus of nursing. I must first take seriously the normative practices that I encounter when somebody nurses; I must precisely describe what actually happens in this situation. My phenomenological approach aims primarily at a description of the *phenomenon* of care. Emphasis is placed first and foremost on the phenomenon, which is why the approach is to be characterised as phenomenological. Only once I have such a description, only once I have such a phenomenology, so to speak, can I begin—in a much later step—to comment on these practices from a normative standpoint.

This phenomenological approach will be of key significance for the interpretation of care as an existential pattern of my method of dealing with reality. This pattern is to be understood in a proto-ethical manner, and not, as is often the case in care ethics, as something that is in itself, in a normative sense, good.

After the phenomenological beginning, I will attempt to apply the phenomenology of care to nursing.

The General Phenomenology of Care

Care is always initiated by an *appeal.* Something appeals to us—perhaps purely coincidentally. I then allow this appeal to become a matter of my *concern.* In accordance with this concern, I develop a *volition*: I *want* that which promotes the thriving—even to the smallest extent—of that which has appealed to us, that which concerns us, regardless of how I may establish what that entails. Eventually I take *practical* action. This connection is what I refer to as care.[2]

Perhaps I hold on to the object of my care in the future and the care becomes love (Freter 2016, pp. 351–363), or perhaps, as the case may also be, I immediately release the source of the appeal from my care again and send it on its way.

In the following section, I will attempt to show how this basic phenomenological structure can indeed be derived from a famous literary account, namely the "Gospel According to Luke", in the so-called Parable of the Good Samaritan.

I will examine this parable as a literary narrative and interpret it without regard to its theological and polemical content. I will concentrate solely on the phenomenon of care, which appears in the text, somewhat inadvertently, as a by no means exclusively Christian phenomenon, but rather as a human phenomenon in general.

Thus it is found in Luke: "[31] And by chance [κατὰ συγκυρίαν; Accidit autem]" (Luke 10, 31)—here there is the moment of coincidence—"there came down a certain priest that way: and when he saw him" (Luke 10, 31)—"him" refers to a person ("ἄνθρωπός τις" (Luke 10, 30)) who had been beaten half to death ("ἡμιθανῆ" (Luke 10, 30)) by robbers—, so when he "saw [ἰδὼν. viso] him, he passed by on the other side [ἀντιπαρῆλθεν. praeterivit]" (Luke 10, 31). The priest saw—"ἰδὼν"—the person in need, but he did not accept the appeal, for whatever reason (Zimmermann 2007, p. 544).[3] He avoided the possible appeal, he does not *want*, in the literal Greek translation, *to go too close* (cf. Wolter 2008, p. 396): "ἀντιπαρῆλθεν", which is made up of ἀντι (not)—παρ (near)—ἔρχομαι (go). This is repeated with a Levite: "[32]And likewise a Levite, when he was at the place, came and looked on him [ἰδὼν. videret] and passed by on the other side [ἀντιπαρῆλθεν. praetereo]" (Luke 10, 32).

Now the Samaritan appears:

> [33] But a certain Samaritan, as he journeyed, came where he was [ἦλθεν κατ' αὐτὸν. venit secus eum]; and when he saw him [ἰδὼν. videns], he had compassion *on him* [ἐσπλαγχνίσθη. misericordia motus est],
> [34] And he went to *him* [προσελθὼν. approprians]. (Luke 10, 33)

The Samaritan does not pass by, but goes to the helpless man—"προσελθὼν"—and is "moved within", σπλαγχνίζομαι, as the original Greek puts it. He was touched, in accordance with the etymology of this verb, in the "innards", in the σπλάγχνα (cf. Frisk 1972, pp. 769 ff.; Zimmermann 2007, p. 539).

The Samaritan, for whatever reason this was possible for him, allowed himself to be appealed to. He makes the injured man his concern and can *come near* (προσέρχομαι) him. To the injured man, to whom he had just now been a stranger—just a "ἄνθρωπός τις"—, the Samaritan becomes the closest (πλησίος, proximus (cf. Luke 10, 29 and 10, 36 ff.)), and the beaten man simultaneously becomes his closest (cf. Wolter 2008, p. 391).

The Samaritan *does not want* the injured man to continue to be in the state in which he has been: *He does not want that which is.* The concern has been compressed, has been turned into volition, substantiated to a volition: *to a volition for the sake of the concern.* The condition of the injured man *ought* to improve. It *ought*, therefore, to be different. *It ought not to be as it is.* This seems to us to be of decisive importance. The Samaritan takes issue with the situation as he finds it. He sets his will against that which is. This appears to be one important source of the ought: when I posit my will, as it arises from my being, against that which is, when I say: it ought not to be so, but rather how I, for the sake of the other person, want it to be. And this will for the sake of another, I suspect, is a preliminary form of the ought.

Thus the Samaritan takes practical action, and as the story continues, he "bound up his wounds, pouring in oil and wine, and set him on his own beast, and brought him to an inn, and took care of him [καὶ ἐπεμελήθη αὐτοῦ. et curam eius egit]" (Luke 10, 34). The care-giver then releases the nameless man from his care (Zimmermann and Zimmermann 2003, pp. 54–58): "[35]And on the morrow when he departed, he took out two pence, and gave *them* to the host, and said unto him, Take care of him ['Επιμελήθητι αὐτοῦ. Curam illus habe]; and whatsoever thou spendest more, when I come again, I will repay thee" (Luke 10, 35). What may have happened after that is not mentioned, but it is not important for these purposes.

As I stated, the Samaritan does not *want* the continued suffering of the nameless man. I can form such a will—I now move away from the connection to the parable—*because* I want to address the concern of the person who has appealed to us: I place my will in the service of their concern. This will is the central element of the story.

The will is then transformed. This will, which I bring forth in the course of my care, encounters me once again—seemingly foreign, seemingly having become independent—as a demand made to myself.

This ought is by no means to be understood universally. With the help of this "origin story" of the ought, I indeed intend to establish that the ought, at least in one of its forms, at least when close to its very first formation, has unfolded and developed out of my own will: will is encountered again as an ought that is addressed to me. This ought, however, is primarily valid *for me*, although I may also wish it to be valid for others as well. But the most important point here is that first and foremost, I subject myself to an ought that, through the transformation from “I want” to “it should be”, has acquired a quasi-objective character for us.

In the course of the care, through the practical actualisation of my being, I have therefore set to work an ought—as short-lived as this ought may perhaps be—to which I have subsequently committed myself. In the course of the care, therefore, normativity itself, the ought-to-be, has become reality: for the sake of the concern, I have brought forth a will, into the service of which I have then placed myself. And I have done this as if this will were no longer my own. This will has seemingly become a will that is addressed to us, meaning: it has become a demand, it has become an ought.

I thus understand an ought as a will that is addressed to us. The ought—at least in this form—can be grasped as something that was once my own volition, a volition that has quasi-extricated itself from us, has transcended us, in order then to encounter us once more as this extricated, transcended volition, addressing us with this will (cf. Freter 2016, pp. 361–363).[4]

I have posited with the ought a *fact*, or to be more precise, an *existential fact* (cf. Freter 2016, pp. 52–59). I have created something new, something that was not there before, a normative entity. And I have subsequently committed myself to this positing—which is entirely my own but at the same time entirely foreign. I can thus newly define care altogether: caring means to believe that one is subject to an ought.

At this point I must point out that the person who cares is by no means restricted to the notion of altruism. It is not to be assumed that somebody who cares has only the well-being of the other person in mind. I in fact suspect that that which I understand as evil actually arises from precisely this pattern of care which I have described here, namely when I only allow myself to be appealed to by myself and place myself exclusively in the service of caring for myself, that is when I care excessively only for myself.[5]

But let us return to the topic at hand: care, as I wish to pinpoint once again, is realised through the quartet of *appeal, concern, volition and practice*. The care-giver wants that to be which promotes the care for the sake of the concern, and in following this takes practical action.

Appeal in the Nursing Context

Care is initiated, as I have found, by an appeal, an appeal which may be directed purely coincidentally towards us. I also find an appeal at the initiation of nursing. However, this appeal has been stripped of any coincidence, and, moreover, at the initiation of nursing, I find the will to allow oneself to be appealed to, the will to encounter the person who wishes to appeal, indeed who must appeal. Nursing thus begins with the nursing care-giver placing him/herself in a position in which he or she can and may be found and approached in this role (cf. Martin et al. 2015, p. 635).[6]

Within this fact, I believe, is contained a first fundamental principle of nursing. The *Principle of the Appeal* states: the nursing care-giver wishes to communicate his or her approachability—in a certain environment at a certain time, and not any longer once these limits of place and time are exceeded. The nursing care-giver wishes to be found in precisely this role (cf. Eley et al. 2010, pp. 10 ff.; 2012, p. 1553[7]; Price 2009, p. 16[8]; Smith and Godfrey 2002; Smith et al. 2013).

I am speaking about what the nursing care-giver "wishes", not what he or she "should" do, for I am not concerned with creating instructions for those who do not wish to nurse, but rather with attempting to understand the (self-produced) ought, the demands to which the person who wishes to nurse—tacitly—subjects him/herself. Subjecting him/herself to these demands is what allows the nursing care-giver to be recognised as such—even when these demands can sometimes not be met, as may be the case in periods of tiredness, overwork or stress.[9]

Normative Uncertainties

In the course of my considerations on the appeal in the nursing context, I have made two claims. Firstly: *nursing is a form of care*. As I have shown though, the care for the well-being of the patient becomes an obligation for the care-giver. This means that secondly: the nursing care-giver acts first and foremost normatively (cf. Bishop and Scudder 1991, p. 18[10]; Smith and Godfrey 2002, p. 302[11]), as he or she works towards *realising that which ought to be for the sake of the patient*, that is: he or she aims to create, maintain, improve or restore a patient's well-being.

Because this is the purpose, that is *realising that which ought to be for the sake of the patient*, ethical problems will *necessarily* arise while nursing. This is due to the fact that the determination of that which ought to be, that which ought to be for the sake of the patient, is—as countless social debates have shown—something which must be repeatedly determined anew. This, however, is the decisive reason to nobilitate nursing as an originary normative practice: the nursing care-giver places him/herself—whether fully aware of this or not—personally as a care-giver (cf. Smith and Godfrey 2002) into the highly contentious field of normative fluctuation—both individual and of society as a whole. This service, it seems to us, does not yet receive the social acknowledgement it deserves (cf. Lachmann 2012, p. 114[12]; Swanson 1993, p. 354).

I have to accept that nursing means exposing oneself to normative uncertainties. Here, as in life in general, there is no ultimate protection from the constant threat of the return of normative obscurity: the well-being of the patient is indeed a very murky subject. The uncertainty of this stipulation, even though it is and must remain an undisputed guideline, shows us that it is of paramount importance—from a normative perspective, which is all that concerns us here—to provide support to care-givers in making decisions, rather than simply handing down instruction manuals and rules and so on that—supposedly—list what is right and wrong.[13]

Let us imagine a patient with diabetes mellitus who refuses to curtail his consumption of sweets. It is indeed *not* unequivocally clear, provided I do not allow myself to be drawn into some form of reductionism, what is to be done in this case. It is not of genuine assistance simply to inform the patient about the course of diabetic illnesses when foodstuffs containing sugar are consumed—although such knowledge is without a doubt necessary for a serious confrontation with the problem. Certainly from such a (reductionist) perspective, it is absolutely necessary to remove access to the foodstuffs in question; however a care-giver may manage this. But, the patient is not simply diabetes mellitus, he is not simply this one disease. He *is* someone who *has* this disease: he *is* someone who *is* also much more than this, namely his entire body, and not only this body inasmuch as diabetes mellitus can be observed within it. He *is* someone who also *has* so much more, for example an attitude regarding his own illness. My patient could—with good reason—insist upon having a short, enjoyable life rather than a long one marked by deprivation

It cannot be clearly decided, if I am to remain within this simple dichotomy, whether the shorter or the longer life is objectively preferable. Objectivity cannot be achieved here. One can argue with good reason in favour of the one option, and with equally good reason in favour of the other. In this situation, the care-giver, despite recourse to supervision and the necessary specialist knowledge and so on, is nevertheless faced with a very personal normative challenge. Furthermore, and this fact must be given recognition, he or she must be given leeway for this decision appropriate to the vagueness of the issue: the solution is not to prescribe one course of action or another, to demand either forced withdrawal or an ignoring of the consumption. It must be possible for the care-giver to make a decision as to the course of action, to create, maintain, improve or restore the patient's well-being.

I have stated firstly: *nursing is a form of care*. This means secondly: nursing is *a* form of care. It is *one particular form* of care, or to be more precise: *nursing is a particular normative human reaction to the notorious frailty of one's neighbour*.

Nursing does *not* accept the (actuated) reality, as it is, as the best possible scenario, but rather attempts—healing, soothing, assisting—to make the best *possible* scenario (*possibilitas*)—I are painfully aware of the darkness surrounding this term—become *reality (actualitas)*. This best possible scenario, always in terms of the patient's needs, can materialise in divergent ways: perhaps in recovery, perhaps in a peaceful death, perhaps in something else.

Because nursing is concentrated in this way, because nursing is adapted in this way to a certain domain—even if that is difficult to define—I can speak of nursing as *accommodated care*. To nurse, I can say, is to care in a very specific way, in an accommodated fashion.[14]

Concern, Volition and Practice in the Nursing Context

If nursing is to be understood as care, it is thus to be presumed that the quaternary phenomenology of care—that is not only the appeal, as I have attempted to show, but also concern, volition and practice—is similarly reflected in nursing.[15] I now wish to conclude my investigation with a brief look at where the reflections of concern, volition and practice in the context of nursing can be found.

Just as the nursing care-giver wishes to be appealed to, he or she subsequently wishes every appeal to become his or her concern. The care accommodated to become nursing is concerned with that which has appealed to it. The *Principle of Concern* states: the nursing care-giver wishes to be concerned with that which was allowed to make the appeal. An appeal is not only noted, but also made a cause for concern.

This cause for concern manifests itself in the direct *volition* to *do* something for the sake of the source of the appeal. The *Principle of Volition and Practice in Nursing* thus states: the nursing care-giver wishes to take practical action for the sake of the concern.

Notes

1. When, in the following discourse, we speak of nursing, we are referring not to the profession of nursing in the narrow sense, but rather to medical practice in its entirety. A compact overview of widespread nursing theories in the narrow sense (Virginia Henderson, Dorothea Orem, Nancy Roper, Monika Krohwinkel, Erwin Böhm) can be found in Lauf (2013, pp. 61–71).

2. Joan Tronto has provided a somewhat similar representation from a feminist-political perspective (cf. Tronto 1993). There are, however, several differences to our approach, particularly the fact that for Tronto, compassion with the other person and the understanding of care as a collective process play an important role. This is not the case in our proto-ethical approach, which is why we will not go into Tronto's work in more detail here. A critical study of the fundamental aspects of Tronto's approach is provided by Edwards (2009, pp. 233–238), an overview to different concepts of care (including Tronto's approach) is provided by Kohlen and Kumbruck (2008).
3. Carl Amery undertook the interesting exercise of allowing the "minor characters" of the parable (the priest, the Levite, the innkeeper and even the leader of the robbers) to express themselves and to explain their respective actions (cf. Amery 1973).
4. It seems, as we wish to note only in passing, to be immaterial for the significance of the ought whether it was created as an existential factum, as we claim here, or whether it encountered me as a facticity.
5. Protest against the tendency of caring ethics to interpret care fundamentally as something essentially good—an idea brought forth primarily by Carol Gilligan and Nel Noddings—has also arisen within the field of nursing studies, cf. for example Allmark (1995); Bradshaw (1996); Edwards (2009, pp. 232 ff).
6. "Care is an affectively charged and selective mode of attention that action, affection, or concern at something, and in effect, it draws attention away from other things. In practice, a person who cares is one who has already chosen an object to care about. Consider, however, that prior to securing a thing to care for, a person must have the capacity or willingness to respond, to be called into action, to be hailed by that object or phenomenon. In short, a person who cares must first be willing and available *to be moved by* this other."
7. "[T]here was notable consistency between students and nurses in reasons for entering nursing affected by neither age nor level of experience. This finding along with high levels of innate personal traits that are conducive to a caring and cooperative nature suggests that individuals are drawn to nursing for similar reasons. There was a general consensus by participants that 'all sorts of personalities make a good nurse' and the dominant trait of a good nurse is that 'desire to care'."

8. "Despite individual differences in perspectives of nurses and nursing, most studies [analysed in this meta-study] identified that nurses held some construction of an 'ideal' nurse that usually focused on caring."
9. The problem of care-givers not being able to meet the necessary demands (e.g. due to a high workload) is mentioned repeatedly in empirical investigations (cf. Price 2009, pp. 16 ff. (on the paradox of caring); Eley et al. 2010, 2012).
10. "Nursing is a practice with an inherent moral sense."
11. "Nursing is by nature a moral endeavour."
12. "Care can be considered simply an ethical task and thus a burden of one more thing to do, or it can be considered a commitment to attending to and becoming enthusiastically involved in the patient's needs."
13. See the contribution by Opgenhaffen in this volume (Chapter "Regulation as an Obstacle to Care? A Care-Ethical Evaluation of the Regulation on the Use of Seclusion Cells in Psychiatric Care in Flanders (Belgium)").
14. There can, of course, also be other accommodations of care, but that is not of interest to me here.
15. Moreover, if nursing is recognised as care, it seems necessary to support and encourage it as care, and consequently to support and encourage the realisation of the constitutive moments of that care—appeal, concern, volition and practice.

References

The English text of the Gospel according to Luke is quoted from:

Carroll, R., & Prickett, S. (Eds.). (2008). *The Bible. Authorized King James Version*. Oxford: Oxford University Press.

The Greek and Latin texts from the Gospel according to Luke are quoted from:

Nestle, E., & Aland, K. (1984). *Novum Testamentum. Graece et Latine* (26th ed.). Stuttgart: Deutsche Bibelgesellschaft.

Allmark, P. (1995). Can There Be an Ethics of Care? *Journal of Medical Ethics, 21*, 19–24.

Amery, C. (1973). Nebenfiguren. In W. Jens (Ed.), *Der barmherzige Samariter* (pp. 19–28). Stuttgart: Kreuz.

Bishop, A. H., & Scudder, J. R. (1991). *Nursing. The Practice of Caring.* New York: National League for Nursing Press.

Bradshaw, A. (1996). Yes! There Is an Ethics of Care: An Answer for Peter Allmark. *Journal of Medical Ethics, 22*, 8–15.

Edwards, S. (2009). Three Versions of an Ethics of Care. *Nursing Philosophy, 10*(4), 231–240.

Eley, R., Eley, D., & Rogers-Clark, C. (2010). Reasons for Entering and Leaving Nursing: An Australian Regional Study. *Australian Journal of Advanced Nursing, 28*(1), 6–13.

Eley, D., Eley, R., Bertollo, M., & Rogers-Clark, C. (2012). Why Did I Become a Nurse? Personality Traits and Reasons for Entering Nursing. *Journal of Advanced Nursing, 68*(7), 1546–1555.

Freter, B. (2016). *Wirklichkeit und existentiale Praxis. Vorarbeiten zu einer Phänomenologie der Normativität entwickelt an narrativen Texten der altgriechischen, neutestamentlichen, mittelhochdeutschen und klassischen deutschen Literatur*. Berlin: Lit-Verlag.

Frisk, H. (1972). *Griechisches etymologisches Wörterbuch. Band 2.* Heidelberg: Carl Winter.

Kohlen, H., & Kumbruck, C. (2008). Care-(Ethik) und das Ethos fürsorglicher Praxis (Literaturstudie). *artec-paper 151*. Retrieved March 22, 2016, from http://nbn-resolving.de/urn:nbn:de:0168-ssoar-219593

Lachman, V. D. (2012). Applying the Ethics of Care to Your Nursing Practice. *Ethics, Law and Policy, 21*, 112–116.

Lauf, U. (2013). Berufskunde. In B. Hein (Ed.), *Altenpflege konkret. Pflegetheorie und -praxis* (pp. 1–93). Urban & Fischer: München.

Martin, A., Myers, N., & Viseu, A. (2015). The Politics of Care in Technoscience. *Social Studies of Science, 45*, 625–641.

Price, S. L. (2009). Becoming a Nurse: A Meta-Study of Early Professional Socialization and Career Choice in Nursing. *Journal of Advanced Nursing, 65*(1), 11–19.

Smith, K. V., & Godfrey, N. S. (2002). Being a Good Nurse and Doing the Right Thing: A Qualitative Study. *Nursing Ethics, 9*(3), 301–312.

Smith, R., Lagarde, M., Blaauw, D., Goodman, C., English, M., Mullei, K., Pagaiya, N., Tangcharoensathien, V., Erasmus, E., & Hanson, K. (2013).

Appealing to Altruism: An Alternative Strategy to Address the Health Workforce Crisis in Developing Countries? *Journal of Public Health, 35*(1), 164–170.

Swanson, K. M. (1993). Nursing as Informed Caring for the Well-Being of Others. *Image: The Journal of Nursing Scholarship, 25*(4), 352–357.

Tronto, J. C. (1993). *Moral Boundaries. A Political Argument for an Ethic of Care.* New York: Routledge.

Wolter, M. (2008). *Das Lukasevangelium.* Tübingen: Mohr Siebeck.

Zimmermann, R. (2007). Berührende Liebe (Der barmherzige Samariter) Lk 10,30-35. In R. Zimmermann (Ed.), *Kompendium der Gleichnisse Jesu* (pp. 538–555). Darmstadt: Wissenschaftliche Buchgesellschaft.

Zimmermann, R., & Zimmermann, M. (2003). Der barmherzige Wirt. Das, Samaritergleichnis‘ (Lk 10,25-37) und die Diakonie. In A. Götzelmann (Ed.), *Diakonische Kirche – Anstöße zur Gemeindeentwicklung und Kirchenreform. Festschrift für Theodor Strohm zum 70. Geburtstag* (pp. 44–58). Heidelberg: Winter.

Open Access This chapter is licensed under the terms of the Creative Commons Attribution 4.0 International License (http://creativecommons.org/licenses/by/4.0/), which permits use, sharing, adaptation, distribution and reproduction in any medium or format, as long as you give appropriate credit to the original author(s) and the source, provide a link to the Creative Commons license and indicate if changes were made.

The images or other third party material in this chapter are included in the chapter's Creative Commons license, unless indicated otherwise in a credit line to the material. If material is not included in the chapter's Creative Commons license and your intended use is not permitted by statutory regulation or exceeds the permitted use, you will need to obtain permission directly from the copyright holder.

Fundamentals of an Ethics of Care

Giovanni Maio

Care: Connecting Virtue and Practice

The ethics of care, or care ethics, developed in the field of bioethics, primarily in response to the lack of context and the rationalist approach of principlism. Care ethics takes an approach which consciously distances itself from principlism and the idea that ethical problems can be solved by means of abstract principles and instead develops its own concepts. What, then, are the specific characteristics of care ethics? The starting point for the formulation of an ethics of care was undoubtedly the book *In a Different Voice* (1982) by Carol Gilligan. In this book Gilligan pursues a theory of "two views of morality" and defines care as a specifically female virtue or disposition. Until now care ethics has thus been seen above all in its relation to feminist ethics, raising the issue of the relationship between care and so-called female morals. This restrictive definition in terms of an "ethics of gender" is not of great help in respect of the medical-ethical

G. Maio (✉)
Department of Medical Ethics and the History of Medicine,
University of Freiburg, Freiburg, Germany

© The Author(s) 2018
F. Krause, J. Boldt (eds.), *Care in Healthcare*,
https://doi.org/10.1007/978-3-319-61291-1_4

Table 1 Tronto's four-phase model with the corresponding ethical elements of an ethics of care, modified according to Conradi (2001)

Phases of care	Ethical elements
1. Recognition of need (caring about)	1. Attentiveness
2. Willingness to respond to (take care of) a need	2. Responsibility
3. Direct action (care-giving)	3. Competence
4. Reaction to the care process (of the care receiver)	4. Responsiveness

implications. It seems more important to reflect instead on the basic characteristics of care ethics, for example on the necessity, underlined by Gilligan, of being there for a person in order to realise care, on her emphasis on the network of relationships that binds us to others, and on the primacy of inner judgement and the personal approach, instead of external obligations. Gilligan's radicalised shift of focus to inner judgement and the personal approach provoked direct criticism and brought out alternative voices. For example, the political scientist Joan Tronto understands care not primarily as virtue, but rather as practice (Tronto 1993); she makes it clear that care cannot be achieved through good intentions alone, but can only be considered to have been carried out when these good intentions have actually resulted in some kind of effect on the other person (Table 1). Tronto thus developed a four-phase model of care:

A model such as this is initially illuminating, because it locates care in connection with attitude and action, with outlook and deeds. But such lists (which are not entirely free of trivialities) cannot hide the fact that they are unable to replace theory or methodical reflection. There is a lot to be said for understanding care ethics not so much as a method unto itself but as something that brings a specific point of view to situations and problems. An example of this deeper reflection can be found in Paul Ricœur.

Care According to Paul Ricœur

In his late work *Oneself as Another*, Paul Ricœur defines care explicitly as a part of humans' ethical duty. He neatly summarises the content of care when he stresses that care is about being "with the other and for them".

He thus understands care in one sense as interaction with the other and at the same time as referring to them. This double reference brings together the two essential aspects of care. Drawing on the Aristotelian concept of friendship, Ricœur focuses on the fact that care is grounded in reciprocity. He thus categorically rejects Emmanuel Levinas' one-sided appeal to care that extends from the other to us, underlining the reciprocity of the care relationship. Care is not oriented in one direction towards the person who receives care. The person providing care also changes as a result. By confronting the unfamiliarity of the care receiver, the care provider expands their own horizons. It is thus care that enables them to find their own identity in unfamiliarity. In care, what was previously seen as self-evident as well as one's view of the world and the self—made one-sided through routine—are broken down and exposed. According to Ricœur, care has a mediating function in that the care provider, in order to really show care, must enter "foreign ground", become distanced from themself, in order to be able to broaden their own standpoint and vantage point.[1] Ricœur thus makes an original connection which goes beyond the link between care and finding one's personal identity to also connect care to the valuable asset of self-esteem: our image of ourselves is formed above all through dialogue with others. By providing care for the other, our own self gains a layer of unfamiliarity, which helps us not only to see ourselves more clearly but also to value ourselves more. At the same time, for Ricœur, caring is always linked to a recollection of our own vulnerability, and this reminder, in which we experience ourselves as being "related" to the person in need of help, triggers a process of change in the giver. Thus through the simple fact of making their need for help known, the care receiver becomes the giver by opening up the care provider to experiences that would otherwise have been denied to them. The awareness of being "related" or "similar" (as Ricœur also says) to the person receiving care, in connection with the fundamental attitude that there is a "reversibility" of the roles in the provision of care, leads to an effort to compensate for the obvious asymmetry and create equality. For Ricœur, care is thus a crucial motivator in the "search for equality in the midst of inequality" (Ricœur1992, p. 192). It represents a call for increased equality, for the abolition of one-sided thinking, and for the facilitation of reciprocity. In pursuing these goals, an inner identification with the other and "the shared admission of fragility" are needed (Ricœur1992, p. 192).

For Ricœur, care is thus a reciprocal phenomenon, because it is only realised when a response is given—that is through the reference to a demand—which in turn depends on active questioning and on a response supported by kindness and consideration. Ricœur describes this response to the other's requirement as a fundamental willingness, "by which the self makes itself available to others" (Ricœur1992, p. 168). He also defines this process of making oneself available and the related openness to the particular nature of the other as a disposition to kindness (Ricœur 1992, p. 189). This disposition lies at the heart of care. The other can initiate a new situation and self-esteem, so long as the care provider is sensitive to the demand that they have made. Ricœur calls the acceptance of the associated responsibility "striving for the good of the other".

At one point, Ricœur also expresses this conception of care in connection with the concept of "benevolent spontaneity", making it clear that care is an interaction which must be supported by a certain fundamental disposition: the disposition of goodwill. Ricœur thus links his conception of care back to motivational contents and emotional factors which present themselves in the immediacy of the interaction with the person in need of care. Care is hence conceived of as a combination of (1) reflexivity (self-awareness), (2) intentionality (being oriented towards the other), (3) affectivity (goodwill), and (4) spontaneity (immediacy).

Systematics of the Core Elements of an Ethics of Care

Now that we have drawn on Paul Ricœur to discuss one of the most well-founded conceptions of care, our focus will turn to developing a more general understanding of care ethics. We have seen that there certainly are differing conceptions, but, all differences aside, a closer look reveals some underlying characteristics which can shed light on the particular nature of care ethics.

Anthropology of Dependence

A central feature of care ethics is the anthropology on which it is based. This anthropology was originally developed as a counterreaction to a form of ethics that (like the principlism described here) focuses on the individual as a sovereign being with the right to self-defence. Care ethics does not, of course, negate the need to respect these rights, but rests upon a different view of humanity. Rather than on the sovereignty of each individual, it focuses on their fundamental dependence. Practising care ethics means recognising that each individual lives within a basic structure of dependence, whether or not they are conscious of this dependence (which was also Gilligan's basic idea). Care ethics thus takes as its point of departure an awareness of the asymmetry of the situation in which people in need of help or care find themselves. Their situation is not so much based on reciprocity but on a reflection of a fundamental state of dependence inherent to all human beings. And it is also this situation that makes care necessary as a form of action constituting a response to this fundamental trait of dependence. What distinguishes care ethics, however, is not just that it acknowledges asymmetry and thus dependence. It also frees this dependence from its negative connotations: from the perspective of care ethics, needing help is not considered an imperfection, but rather something normal and generally paradigmatic for relationships.

In this context, asymmetry does not refer to the cementing of a benevolent paternalism. Instead, it concerns the recognition that although the situation may be one of inequality, this does not negate the postulate of an equal level of respect and of equality between people. In other words, an ethics of care acknowledges the different degrees of sovereignty that a person may have in their particular situation, but without relativising on any level the fundamental equality of all humans in their moral rights and relationships of recognition. Its ultimate aim (as we saw with Ricœur) is instead, at the same time, to balance out the asymmetry of sovereignty by means of the equality of the people involved.

Being in Relationships

Relationships play a crucial role in care ethics in three regards. Firstly, they are based on a concept of anthropology that does not just perceive humans as dependent beings but also interprets them as beings oriented towards relationships with other humans. Relationships are a fundamental feature of human existence. Secondly, relationships are seen as playing a significant role in the development of ethical problems, particularly with regard to a lack of relationships. For care ethics, relationships thus become a prism through which to view ethical problems. Finally, relationships are also a crucial strategy for resolving such conflicts. Against this background it is clear why care ethics makes reference to the crucial importance of human connectedness in resolving ethical problems. This relational approach to ethics also involves an appreciation of other virtues that have a stabilising effect on relationships, such as forbearance and forgiveness or devotion and trust. Care ethics thus places significantly more value on affective connections and prioritises interactive actions for resolving ethical conflicts.

However, since promoting relationships as a solution to every problem would not be appropriate either, a nuanced approach is required here. It is not unusual for the entanglement in relationships itself to cause problems for patients, for example when they find themselves in a situation of dependence and need help extracting themselves in order to resolve the problem. For the people providing help, this focus on relationships is also always a balancing act, since they must guard against becoming too emotionally involved and ultimately burning themselves out. This is where we begin to see the limits of expecting too much of relationships when it comes to providing solutions. Nonetheless, the emphasis on the moral dimension of relationships and the appreciation of virtues which make relationships more stable are two of the crucial elements at the heart of an ethics of care.

Being Situation-Oriented

A key issue with regard to care ethics is that of the reason or justification for a particular action or reaction. While principlism adopts a deductive approach here, deriving action from abstract principles (and justifying it by way of these principles), care ethics takes a fundamentally different path. Rather than basing its actions on an abstract rule and moving from here to practice, it takes practice itself as the foundation for selecting the action required. It thus does not follow a deductive model, but instead sees the immediacy and singularity of a particular situation as an instruction to decide on the action that seems most appropriate in that situation. Thus, while principlism applies rules, care ethics is concerned with a fitting response that must be developed based on the situation, since the specific nature of a situation cannot be confronted adequately simply by applying rules. This shows that, in terms of method alone, care ethics is not concerned with the criterion of generalisability or with a Kantian idea of universalism; rather, it focuses on understanding the particular and incomparable nature of the patient and their situation. Generalisability is replaced by singularity and particularity. This is reminiscent of hermeneutic ethics insofar as the particular point of view of care ethics lies specifically in inquiring into the particular and thus the unique nature of the other. It is therefore no coincidence that the hermeneutist Ricœur of all people advocates an ethics of care, nor that—drawing on the Aristotelian concept of phronesis—he identifies "practical wisdom" as the methodical basis for ethical judgements. Ricœur wanted care to be understood as a guarantee that the unique nature of the other is protected against being taken over by generalising postulates. He sees the fundamental role of care in saving the otherness of the other.

In summary, this aspect of situational specificity can be divided into three elements:

(a) emphasis on immediacy and acknowledgement of immediate perception
(b) recognition of the singularity of the situation
(c) need for a creative resolution to conflict rather than one that is simply rule-based.

Care ethics thus represents a progressive alternative to simple instrumental rationality.

Responsiveness

In the light of the above, the distinguishing feature of care ethics is that it is defined less by initiative than by responsiveness. It responds or reacts to the needs of the person who is dependent on help. Care ethics is primarily response-focused. It is the other who calls for care. Thus care ethics is linked to the attitude and gestures of "turning to" somebody and necessitates the capacity to approach the other. This requires an attitude of listening, of receptiveness, of understanding, essentially of close attention. Here, too, we can see a similarity with hermeneutic ethics, although care ethics involves more than just understanding; it contains the impulse to change, to realise care (Maio 2015). This impulse to realise care can be understood as the impulse to implement the response we are urged to give by the urgent situation of the other. In this context, Emmanuel Levinas defined care as "being called on" by the other.

Accepting the Indefinable

As care ethics does not aim to be rule-based and instead takes the specific situation as its point of departure, the demand made on the result of the ethical judgement is also entirely different. Ethics based on deductive reasoning demands exactitude and unambiguousness, following the motto: Is this permitted or not permitted? Required or not required? Right or wrong? Care ethics does not apply these categories, which constitutes another similarity with hermeneutic ethics. Instead, it is characterised by a tolerance for ambiguity; as it takes seriously the specific features of each situation, it cannot predict what is right and what is wrong. A situation may remain ambivalent until the last moment. But care ethics does not see ambivalence as a state that should be abolished by any means—paying attention to, allowing and bearing ambivalence are part and parcel of the methodical approach of an ethics of care. In other words: from the epistemology of particularity comes an acceptance of ambiguity. There is no one correct solution, but rather a spectrum of solutions; there is no single right answer, but rather what is appropriate in each case, and there is also no objective solution that is connected with a universalistic pretension. Instead, it is a case of the particular and thus the always fallible.

Giving Preference to Emotional Knowledge

The above criteria show that care ethics differs from other forms of ethics above all in the way in which problems are perceived. It perceives the ethical problem in different terms, which are not just related to the above basic elements, but rest more fundamentally on a wider concept of knowledge. For care ethics, knowing the objectifiable and formalisable facts does not suffice; care ethics also draws on what could be called "implicit knowledge". The critical role of relationships, the demand for an adequate perception of the situation, and the prioritising of creative solutions over deductive inference necessitate implicit forms of knowledge such as experiential knowledge, situational knowledge, and relationship knowledge. Valuing these forms of knowledge, which go beyond the confines of a formal-logical approach, is the essence of care ethics. They are forms of knowledge that cannot be learnt by heart but must be practised. According to care ethics, competence could be described as skill in dealing with ambiguity. The ability to cope with complexity plays a significantly more constitutive role here than in other forms of ethics. This perhaps also explains why the medical community continues to give little importance or support to care ethics. Care ethics represents a counterpoint to operational rationality because it practices a rationality of its own, in which feelings, intuition, and sensations are just as important as calculations, and in which experience is ascribed an epistemological value which is overlooked in the structural logic of modern medicine.

In this regard, care ethics is more progressive than many forms of principlism, because it does away with the prejudice of the irrationality of feeling, because it takes the knowledge content of feelings seriously and in this respect constitutes an implicit plea to place more value on emotional knowledge. The specific challenge of care ethics, on the other hand, is to take this emotional knowledge seriously in such a way that it is not set in opposition to cognitive knowledge. A healthy balance must be struck between both forms of knowledge, placing more value on emotional knowledge as a creative factor while cognitive knowledge remains present in the same way as a constant check and balance. Care ethics can only truly bear fruit when it draws on emotional knowledge to enable unique and creative approaches without being absolved of the obligation to justify such creative solutions with transparent and comprehensible arguments.

Giving Preference to Space for Growth

Care ethics does not just expand the above-described form of knowledge and insights; its core elements also open up an alternative view of how to deal with ethical problems. Where the focus of care ethics lies in perceiving the complexity of an ethical problem, and where this complexity or ambiguity necessitates a more receptive approach, the response to the problem will also be evaluated using entirely different criteria than those used when focusing on structural functionality. There is a similarity to hermeneutic ethics here in that it is not rapid, confident action that counts, but rather a tentative and considerate approach. This entails a different definition of good actions, one where the guiding values are careful reflection and prudence. It was Carol Gilligan herself, the initiator of the care ethics debate, who emphasised hesitation and tentative consideration as indicators of care, and, as we saw above, Paul Ricœur also talks explicitly of consideration. Precisely because care ethics assumes that there are no unambiguous solutions, it attributes more value to doubt; the attitude of tentative hesitation has no trace here of the negative connotations that are necessarily attached to it in the constant bustle of large medical institutions. This confers on care ethics nothing short of a subversive power in relation to action as well. This subversive power can be extremely restorative because it can give rise to the insight that good medicine means not simply *doing* things but also allowing these things space to thrive. This praxeology of caution could make it possible to rediscover the value of giving things space to thrive, to mitigate the tendency towards actionism, and to introduce a way of thinking that makes a clearer distinction between medicine (as care) and industry (as production site).

Limits of Care Ethics

It has become clear that care ethics renounces a universalistic pretension and instead turns towards the unique and the particular. It thus constitutes a necessary correction to the prevalent hegemony of the structural-functional approach. However, renouncing universalistic pretensions inevitably raises the objection that care becomes arbitrary and relative. This reproach can only be refuted by making it clear that individual decisions are taken within a predefined framework, which is not invalidated by the particularity of a situation but remains in place as a constitutive framework.

A second criticism has already been discussed above. The fundamental significance that care ethics attributes to relationships and attention also has the potential, in some situations, to place excessive demands both on the treatment team and on the patient. Sometimes a patient has no desire to enter into a relationship, but simply wants to make use of a service. This objection can be fundamentally rejected using care ethics itself, since an ethics of care, understood correctly, should take its specific starting point seriously in such a way that in the case of doubt it recognises that a particular situation requires a distanced approach based more on principlism or ethics of ought. This highlights once again the fact that care ethics represents a very particular approach to ethical problems which cannot and should not be the most appropriate solution to all situations and medical-ethical problems. Care ethics is only as good as the way in which it is applied. It will only be beneficial when it is applied to problems for which it is the most suitable method. In contrast, attempts to elevate it to the level of a medical-ethical paradigm will inevitably result in shortcomings, not in care ethics itself but in the diligence that is applied when choosing it as the method to be used in specific contexts and situations.

Conclusions

Care ethics developed as a reaction to the one-sided thinking of principlism and duty ethics or, as it is sometimes called, ethics of justice. This context has induced polarisation which obscures the fact that both care ethics and principlism are needed. They are not alternative models; they must be allowed to complement one another. In order for medicine to do justice to a patient, there must be an awareness of principles and basic rights and of the significance of a principle as abstract as that of human dignity. That much is indisputable. But on its own it is no guarantee that the patient will truly be helped. In order to help the patient in their specific situation, it is necessary to take a highly individualised approach and develop a strategy that will really help that person. Such a strategy cannot be reduced to adapting rules or limited to subjective arbitrariness. It demands an individual approach to a specific person within a predefined framework. The value of care ethics lies its assumption that the dependence of the other demands the personal acceptance of responsibility. This acceptance of responsibility (the crucial role of the "response" should be borne in mind here) goes beyond ensuring basic rights.

Care ethics, whose core aspects we have highlighted above, thus enriches ethics, makes it more stimulating, and brings to it greater substance that cannot easily be codified. But the specific richness of this substance can only fully develop when it is firmly located within a fixed framework of principles which is not in opposition to care ethics but on the contrary is what finally enables care ethics to be realised. Paul Ricœur neatly summarises this complementary relationship when he emphasises that the power of judgement which is so crucial for care "consists in inventing conduct that will best satisfy the exception required by solicitude, by betraying the rule to the smallest extent possible" (Ricœur 1992, p. 269).

Note

1. Axel Honneth takes a similar approach when, referring to the granting of care, he formulates the possibility of a "decentred perspective" (Honneth, 1996, p. 74).

References

Conradi, E. (2001). *Take Care. Grundlagen einer Ethik der Achtsamkeit*. Frankfurt am Main: Campus.

Gilligan, C. (1982). *In a Different Voice*. Harvard: Harvard University Press.

Honneth, A. (1996). *The Struggle for Recognition: The Moral Grammar of Social Conflicts*. Cambridge: The MIT Press.

Maio, G. (2015). *Den kranken Menschen verstehen. Für eine Medizin der Zuwendung*. Freiburg: Alber.

Ricœur, P. (1992). *Oneself as Another*. (K. Blamey, Trans.). Chicago: University of Chicago Press.

Tronto, J. C. (1993). *Moral Boundaries: A Political Argument for an Ethic of Care*. London: Routledge.

Open Access This chapter is licensed under the terms of the Creative Commons Attribution 4.0 International License (http://creativecommons.org/licenses/by/4.0/), which permits use, sharing, adaptation, distribution and reproduction in any medium or format, as long as you give appropriate credit to the original author(s) and the source, provide a link to the Creative Commons license and indicate if changes were made.

The images or other third party material in this chapter are included in the chapter's Creative Commons license, unless indicated otherwise in a credit line to the material. If material is not included in the chapter's Creative Commons license and your intended use is not permitted by statutory regulation or exceeds the permitted use, you will need to obtain permission directly from the copyright holder.

The Interdependence of Care and Autonomy

Joachim Boldt

Introduction

Since the 1960s, the principle of autonomy has increasingly been hailed as the cornerstone of medical ethics. Today, it is the prime focus of medical ethicists when assessing clinical research trials and therapy decisions at the bedside. Historically, this development is a reaction to scandalous medical research trials on humans in the mid-twentieth century. Experiments on humans in concentration camps in Nazi Germany as well as harmful and racist trials in the USA up to the 1970s clearly indicated that doctors were willing to disregard the will and well-being of individual patients in the name of what they declared to be scientific medical progress.

Apparently, the traditional ethos of the medical profession was not sufficient to prevent aberrations of this sort. The obligation not to perform any therapeutic or research intervention unless the patient is informed

J. Boldt (✉)
Department of Medical Ethics and the History of Medicine,
University of Freiburg, Freiburg, Germany

© The Author(s) 2018

F. Krause, J. Boldt (eds.), *Care in Healthcare*,
https://doi.org/10.1007/978-3-319-61291-1_5

and consents to the procedure was therefore introduced with great emphasis as an important, if not the most important, element of the medical profession's set of ethical norms. Although there were select earlier legal and ethical calls to incorporate patient consent into medical practice, the medical ethos prior to this development was mainly oriented towards not harming patients and, to the extent possible, promoting their well-being. Calls to respect the autonomy of patients thus entered the scene of medicine as part of an ethical orientation that, it was supposed, had not previously been included in the traditional medical ethos of caring for the well-being of patients.

This development has many effects on medical practice today. From an ethical standpoint, there is prima facie nothing wrong with strengthening the rights of patients in the medical encounter. On the contrary, if the traditional medical ethos lacks a focus on patient autonomy, and if medical ethics can help reinforce and justify the importance of patient autonomy, medicine ought to accept this new ethical orientation and incorporate it into its ethos. Most famously, the medical ethicists Beauchamp and Childress took this new orientation into account when setting up their set of biomedical ethical principles (Beauchamp and Childress 2013): Physicians ought to respect patient autonomy. In addition, they ought to minimise harm and maximise well-being, and finally, they ought to strive for the just distribution of scarce resources.

In what is to follow, I will argue that despite appearances, thinking of autonomy as a separate normative principle in addition to caring for well-being suffers from severe ethical drawbacks. What was and still is needed is instead a meaningful interpretation of the interdependence of autonomy and care, not a new principle besides care.

A Conventional Limit to Autonomy in Medicine

Numerous guidelines, regulations, conventions and laws spell out the details of what is implied by respect for autonomy in the medical context. The common understanding is that respecting autonomy entails a patient's right to refuse any medical treatment, regardless of whether the treatment appears medically necessary to restore health or, in the most extreme case, to save the patient's life. The right to autonomy is thus seen as a right of defence. Any medical intervention is an intervention into the patient's body, and no one ought to be allowed to directly intervene in the body of another person unless this person gives consent. At the same time, autonomy in the medical context does not mean that patients have a right to demand medical interventions that are not "medically indicated". That is to say, they cannot request interventions that, from a medical point of view, would not help to restore or maintain health, alleviate pain or suffering, or that would do more harm than good.

For those who presume that ethical rights ought to be consistently organised, this must come as a surprise. If patients are allowed to do harm to themselves by rejecting effective treatment, why should they not, in principle, have the right to request an intervention that does harm to themselves, and only to themselves, provided they are duly informed about any harms and benefits? Obviously, autonomy is counterbalanced in this case by another normative orientation. This orientation is a rudimentary form of the care perspective: Avoid doing harm to others. Although one may have to accept that someone may harm themselves by rejecting offers of help, inflicting harm on another person ought to be avoided, even if the request comes from the person themselves.

In health care, autonomy and care are thus balanced against each other. On the one hand, autonomy constitutes a right of defence against unwanted treatment, even if that treatment would lead to better health. On the other hand, care ensures that no therapeutically unnecessary harm is done to patients, even if they do make a corresponding request, and that medical interventions are restricted to restoring or maintaining health and to alleviating pain and suffering.

The Thrust of the Autonomy Principle

The practicability of these rules and regulations notwithstanding, this is an ethically puzzling situation. Taking John Stuart Mill's influential writings as the root of the current mainstream understanding of the autonomy principle, the basic idea of this principle is that individuals ought to be allowed to do whatever they want as long as their actions do not harm others: "The only freedom which deserves the name, is that of pursuing our own good in our own way, so long as we do not attempt to deprive others of theirs, or impede their efforts to obtain it" (Mill 1869, p. 13).

Autonomy here consists of the right to act in accordance with one's preferences and interests. This right is to be respected as long as carrying out the actions in question does not harm others. Mill assumes that a basic ability to distance oneself from overwhelming emotions, to sort interests, and to take factual information into account is a prerequisite of this right. "Unless he is a child, or delirious, or in some state of excitement or absorption incompatible with the full use of the reflecting faculty" (Mill 1869, chapter 5, p. 5), the freedom of the individual with regard to his or her own good is to be respected.

Now, by itself the autonomy principle does not convey any reason for why it is good to have a specific preference or why it is good to help others to have a preference apart from the fact that this is the other's preference. The autonomy principle does not provide an answer for someone asking themselves whether they should have a certain preference and why, nor does it offer guidance to someone who is in a position to provide support to another person and is wondering whether they should regard that person's preference as worthy of support.

It follows from the autonomy principle that one ought to be allowed to reject medical treatment, even if the treatment is medically advisable. It further follows that attempting to understand and perhaps alter a patient's preferences is unjustified, since the only justification for the preference is the fact that the patient holds this preference. A similar case can be made regarding assisted suicide and voluntary euthanasia. Taking one's own life primarily concerns oneself. Assuming that this act does not compromise the well-being of others, and assuming that one chooses this option as the result of a clear-minded process of reasoning on one's prospects, there is no justification for interfering with or objecting to this choice from the point of view of autonomy. What is more, if a person who is determined to commit suicide does not have the means or opportunity to do so, experts who have the required know-how could be justified in acting on this person's behalf on the basis of respect for autonomy. Asking the patient why he prefers to end his life in order to be able to understand and evaluate this preference must be seen as misguided.

In accordance with this claim, when Mill is concerned with whether one person should be allowed to "counsel" another or "instigate" them to do something, he is not thinking about whether or not it is good, independent of the preferences one happens to have, to act in a certain way. He is concerned instead with whether people should be allowed to counsel others who share a preference that may be met with reproach at a societal level on how to best act in accordance with that preference. For example, should one be allowed to counsel someone who likes gambling on how best to gamble? Mill answers this question in the affirmative, provided the counsellor does not derive a personal benefit from his advice (Mill 1869, chapter 5, p. 8). Accordingly, following Mill, supporting someone else's preference to end their life is justifiable as long as one does not do so for personal gain. Still, and this is the important point, questioning this way of acting from a point of view independent of the preference one happens to have must be seen as pointless and, in addition, unjustifiable if one thereby aims to alter the preferences of the other person.

Assessing Reasons for Doing What One Wants to Do to Oneself

In order to conclude that it is good—not only from the point of view of an individual who has a certain preference but from a point of view independent of given preferences—to act in a certain way, the desired state of affairs must additionally be presumed to be good from some sort of inter-individual standpoint. The term "inter-individual" here is meant to indicate that this point of view must refer to reasons that can appeal to more than just those who happen to have a specific preference. Utilitarian ethics, for example, clearly rests on the assumption that is always possible to supply this kind of inter-individual reason for acting one way rather than another.

The ethical debate concerning enhancement is a case in point. Enhancement is the use of pharmaceuticals and medical technologies by healthy people in order to improve their mental, emotional, or physical abilities. How can enhancing oneself be ethically evaluated? Some individuals may, for example, wish to enhance their ability to stay focussed over long periods of time by using psychiatric drugs; others may not. If one assumes that the consequences of the decision to enhance oneself—or not—are confined to oneself, on the basis of the autonomy principle alone, either preference is valid. In terms of justifying and evaluating this preference, nothing more can be said. If one follows a utilitarian premise, however, it becomes possible to evaluate these preferences on an inter-individual basis. If enhancement serves the interests of more people as compared to non-enhancement, then enhancement ought to be pursued and promoted. Thus, as is usually argued in the enhancement debate, following the utilitarian premise, the basically accidental preference to enhance oneself turns into an ethical, inter-individual obligation. Conversely, this also implies that the autonomous individual decision on whether or not to enhance oneself becomes a choice between courses of action that can be ethically assessed. In the case of a utilitarian assessment, carrying out enhancements would be seen as favourable, as long as the benefit–harm ratio of enhancement is better than that of non-enhancement.

In this way, an inter-individual, reason-providing ethics supplements the autonomy principle with content that guides actions, thereby making it possible to understand and reconstruct what it means to critically assess one's own preferences and those of others. On the basis of the autonomy principle alone, reflecting upon and debating preferences is a pointless undertaking, since in this case there are by definition no inter-individual reasons that could always serve as a shared basis for this reflection. Individuals may agree on a certain preference, but if they do not agree and do not find shared basic interests underlying their diverging preferences, the disagreement cannot be bridged. Supplementing the autonomy principle with a reason-providing ethics thus places all individuals in a shared space of reasons, in which debating preferences and reaching consensus are in principle always possible.

However, introducing a reason-providing ethics can also have negative consequences for autonomy. For example, one of the conundrums of the current enhancement debate is that each individual must be free to choose whether or not he or she wants to make use of these technologies. This is the case in the debate on reproductive enhancement, for example. The term "liberal eugenics" was introduced in this debate in order to highlight that it should be up to individual parents whether their offspring ought to be enhanced.[1] At the same time, when arguments in favour of enhancement are based on utilitarian assumptions, as they often are, it follows that when enhancement results in benefits for the majority, it ought to be obligatory. It has been suggested, for instance, that if an enhancement drug of the future would allow surgeons to save more patients, the use of this drug could be made obligatory for this profession (Greely et al. 2008). In such cases, autonomy gives way to a reason-providing ethics, since nothing can be put forth in defence of autonomy apart from the fact that following ethical, in this case utilitarian, reason may not conform to the will of the individual. Now, changing the will of an individual in accordance with inter-individual reasons is what ethical demands and ethical reasoning are all about. Simply combining the autonomy principle with an inter-individual reason-providing ethics account therefore necessarily weakens autonomy.

No Conception of a Shared Good

These relations highlight an important point. It becomes apparent that the autonomy principle is a non-ethical principle in the sense that it does not provide reasons for acting one way rather than another, provided the act does not directly interfere with the well-being of others. Under these conditions, the autonomy principle can provide no inter-individual reasons for preferring one specific course of action over another. As a correlate, the autonomy principle cannot provide any guidance for decision-making in these cases. The process of will-formation thus appears to be a matter of accident. Whatever comes to be one's interest is what guides one's decisions and must be accepted as such.

Someone who observes behaviour that they find puzzling or wrongheaded is not obliged to interfere, ask for reasons or try to convince the observed actor of the superiority of a different way of behaving. To take up an example provided by John Stuart Mill, if I observe someone who is headed towards a bridge and I know that it will collapse under the person's weight, I am not obliged to interfere, to ask why the person is putting himself into such a dangerous situation or to try to convince him that it would be better to stay away from the bridge. All these interventions would be based on the assumption that my preference not to plummet ought to be the other person's preference as well. However, this is clearly not the case, since the observed person is choosing to step on the bridge. As Mill argues, the only mistake I may presume the person walking is making is that he is not correctly informed about the bridge's condition. If I have provided him with this information and he keeps on walking anyway, further attempts to prevent him from his course of action must be seen as unwarranted interventions into his individual freedom (Mill 1869, chapter 5, p. 5).

The most fundamental way to express these characteristics and implications of the autonomy principle is to say that the autonomy principle does not include a conception of a shared or potentially sharable idea of a good life. Such an idea would justify attempts to understand and discuss reasons for acting one way rather than another. Interests could be understood as preliminary judgements on what ought to be regarded as good, which are then always open to revision. In contrast, following the autonomy principle, one may help others to fulfil their will if one is in a position to do so and if the other person asks for and needs help, regardless of how one assesses these aims oneself. The justification on which this option to help rests is that the end which the other person wants to realise is obviously in their interest and thus promotes what they regard as good for themselves. Conversely, if the person rejects an offer of help, such as a medical treatment, this is what they want, and no further attempts to change the will are called for. Attempts to alter what a person wants are confined to giving factual information. Doing more would have to be seen as unduly influencing the other person's will, since there is no way to understand this exertion of influence as part of what the other person themselves would do or wants to do. Giving reasons for alternative courses of action becomes an unwarranted act of intrusion as soon as these reasons do not refer to the given interests and preferences of the other person. In other words, according to the autonomy principle, reasons for actions are solely the given interests of the acting person. Inter-individual reasons cannot be part of the individual process of will-formation.

The Autonomy Dilemma

The argument so far appears to end in a dilemma. Relying solely on the autonomy principle makes individual decision-making look like a speechless, almost mechanistic, or at least communication free activity. With regard to actions that do not directly harm others, no inter-individual, ethical reflection should make sense. However, if one introduces inter-individual reason-providing ethics accounts in addition to the autonomy principle, these accounts necessarily tend to diminish the validity of autonomy, as the utilitarian reasoning in the enhancement debate shows. As the dilemma stands, one must choose between contingent autonomous will on the one hand and universally prescriptive ethical demands on the other.

Neither of the two alternatives fits very well with how humans actually tend to behave when confronted with individual therapeutic choices that have a significant impact on their future life. Patients can reflect upon such choices together with relatives, friends, or members of their health care team, without thereby sacrificing their autonomy to universal ethical demands. Quite the contrary, this inter-individual reflection on the good life is often the catalyst for truly autonomous choice. What is more, helping someone facing such a choice by supporting them and promising future support is often regarded as ethically valuable rather than as an intrusion into personal freedom. Hence what is needed is a concept of autonomy that can account for these phenomena and thus resolve the autonomy dilemma.

Kant on Autonomy

When looking for alternative concepts of autonomy, Kant's philosophy is a natural place to start. After all, it is Kant who explicitly uses the term "autonomy", whereas Mill, for example, speaks of freedom and individuality instead. For Kant, autonomy is not just the ability to act upon individual preferences and to grasp factual information that has relevance for how to accomplish an end. On the contrary, acting in accordance with one's autonomy for Kant is tantamount to acting ethically. This is because when one reflects on a possible action from the perspective of autonomy, one applies a test of practical reason, that is an ethical test, to this action, namely the test of universalisability. One is supposed to ask oneself whether what one plans to do could be done by everyone "without contradiction" (Kant 1996, p. 75, BA 57). According to Kant, this is a test which one must necessarily accept, because as a practically deliberating person one is part of the realm of universal practical reason, and in this realm, the only ethical criterion that does not rest on contingent preferences is the test of universalisability. Moreover, this test is not imposed on reason and practical reasoners from somewhere else, but originates within reason itself. It is a law that reason and oneself as a reasoner impose upon concrete cases of reason-guided will-formation and decision-making.

For example, refusing to help someone when help could be provided at no great cost to oneself cannot be universalised, according to Kant, since if this preference were a universal law, a situation could arise in which one would need help oneself and not receive it. Hence, Kant concludes that a world in which no one helps others might be thinkable without contradiction, but it cannot be desired without contradiction (Kant 1996, p. 75, BA 56). To take another example, the desire to take one's life when one's future appears to bring more harm than happiness is, following Kant, contradictory, since if everyone adopted this preference, humankind would extinguish itself and there would be no one left to formulate and pursue preferences at all. Therefore, he claims, this preference contradicts its own condition when universalised (Kant 1996, p. 73f, BA 53).

Much has been said for and against these examples and for and against Kant's approach to autonomy and ethics in general. In the context of the discussion here, namely with regard to the autonomy dilemma, Kant's approach initially appears to be a promising way to bring ethical content to the principle of autonomy and to understand will-formation as a reason-guided process. After all, autonomy is thought to involve ethical reasoning. Will-formation and decision-making about one's own future and well-being can be regarded as ethical reason-guided phenomena, as especially the second example above shows. Upon closer scrutiny, however, Kant's approach has serious limitations with regard to resolving the dilemma of ethical content. In order to resolve this dilemma, an account of autonomy is needed. On the one hand, this account must understand will-formation as a process that is guided by ethical reasons. On the other hand, this must be an open process in which certain solutions cannot be flagged as right or wrong without a deliberative, intersubjective exchange. Such an exchange should be held together by a justified sense of having a shared aim, but, at the same time, it must be assumed that right and wrong cannot be inferred from this shared aim without intersubjective deliberation.

Kant's use of the criterion of universalisability points in a different direction. The way in which he treats the question of whether it is ethically justified to take one's life if one's future life does not appear to be worth living is a case in point. He does not imagine this to be a weighing of multiple points of view or a process involving intersubjective social support. Rather he assumes that individually applying the test of universalisability inevitably leads to the conclusion that suicide is not ethically allowed. In other words, the shared aim of acting in accordance with the test of universalisability does not leave room for interpretation or different forms of concretisation in specific contexts as part of a process of intersubjective reason-guided communication.

What is more, critics have pointed out that contrary to Kant's own supposition, planned actions cannot be ethically justified or prohibited on the basis of the criterion of universalisability. These critics claim that Kant relies on implicit hidden assumptions that render planned actions non-universalisable. Therefore, the criterion of universalisability as such is empty. To take the two examples given above, someone who is willing to accept that he will not receive help in cases where he might need it might not see any contradiction if his preference not to help others were universalised. In the same vein, it can be argued that the assumed fact that a preference for suicide, if universalised, undermines the possibility of there being any wills is only a contradiction if one regards the existence of wills as undoubtedly desirable.[2]

It might be possible to save Kant from this criticism and perhaps also to develop an interpretation of his theory that can resolve the autonomy dilemma.[3] However, since there are other philosophical accounts of autonomous will-formation that are better suited to resolve this dilemma from the start, it makes sense to turn to these approaches instead.

Hermeneutic Autonomy

One way to escape the autonomy dilemma is to look for an understanding of individual will-formation that introduces reason and inter-individual reflection as guiding factors in this process, without at the same time assuming a definite set of ethical norms that trump individual choice. Many accounts of the self that have been developed in hermeneutic philosophy can be read in this way.

Most notably, Paul Ricoeur sees will-formation as a reason-guided process. Reasons are not just given preferences. They always include a judgement about what is to be regarded as good in an inter-individual sense. If a certain course of action is judged as being good, any person in a similar situation ought to be able to follow this judgement, regardless of whether or not they initially have such a preference. The judgement need not be restricted to instrumental goodness, according to which an action is good if it serves as a means to bring about a desired state of affairs. "Good" also covers actions of which one assumes that they can be part of what constitutes a "'good life' with and for others, in just institutions" (Ricoeur 1992, p. 172). Therefore, forming one's own will is potentially always an inter-individual, communicative relation and contains a "dialogical dimension" (Ricoeur 1992, p. 180). Recognising and weighing reasons involves taking up the perspective of others. One does not begin decision-making with a fixed set of preferences that just need to be correctly informed in order to lead to what the individual then can regard as a good decision. On the contrary, decision-making starts as an always in principle open search for reasons which are formed by taking up a number of points of view through which one finds one's own perspective.

If this is a correct model of what it means to form a will, a debate about what is good is a seamless extension of the internal will-forming process. In such a debate, each standpoint functions as a reason that must be weighed and assessed, just as reasons and standpoints are internally assessed in the will-forming process. Hence, the result of a debate can have an influence on the individual will, regardless of the standpoint and preferences that made up this individual will in the first place. If someone is convinced by such a debate and changes their will accordingly, this is essentially identical to the process by which one forms one's will oneself.

A pressing question for any such account is how one can settle the issue of what is to be regarded as good in a specific situation. Ricoeur does not assume a fixed set of norms that can help solve this problem, nor should finding a decision be a matter of power or contingency or other factors external to reflection. It is important to adhere to this claim, since otherwise debating the good becomes a matter of prescriptively declaring the good or settling for an arbitrary assumption of what should be regarded as good. One would then find oneself back in the dilemma mentioned above. Hermeneutic ethics thus presupposes a shared orientation towards the good that cannot directly be translated into concrete aims and actions but that nevertheless acts as a transcendent, only partly achievable point of consensus. According to Ricoeur, the ethical orientation towards a good life is just this: a shared orientation which can be assumed to be of universal validity, while its concrete meaning can differ and needs to be determined with regard to context.[4]

It may be helpful to compare this understanding of the notion of the good to the notion of truth in science. In scientific practice, "truth" functions as a universal guiding norm that shapes actions and debates. At the same time, whether one has reached the truth or not can always be called into question. Agreeing that one is looking for the truth thus does not settle arguments about what is to be regarded as true in specific circumstances. Nonetheless, it provides a general and universal aim that guides scientific inquiry and, as such, provides a shared basis for resolving conflict.

Hermeneutic autonomy stresses the procedural and inter-individual character of will-formation and decision-making. Due to this shift of focus, hermeneutic autonomy does not dissolve individual will-formation into contingent autonomous willing, nor does it subject autonomy to a prescriptive, overarching ethical norm that in itself defines what a good will ought to look like. In this way, it escapes the autonomy dilemma.

This kind of an account of autonomy contains the idea of a good which, firstly, need not already be present in the form of given preferences, and which, secondly, can be grasped and shared by exchanging reasons inter-individually. Nonetheless, such an account does rest on non-trivial metaphysical assumptions—as does any theory that incorporates an idea of truth or truth-seeking that is intended to have an effect on action. It is important to be aware of this point, since these metaphysical assumptions are one of the main reasons for objecting to these approaches in philosophical debates.[5] A discussion of these implications must be left aside here, however.

Enabling Autonomy

From this perspective, making up one's mind and acting autonomously does not consist in determining and following contingently given preferences and being equipped with relevant factual knowledge. Rather, forming an autonomous will means taking part in an ongoing dialogue. This dialogue need not be restricted to verbal communication and it need not always take place between co-present interlocutors. Convictions may be expressed nonverbally and affectively, and one may find convincing attitudes and perspectives in books, films or other media. In any case, when forming a will, one is positioning oneself in this dialogue and finding one's own standpoint and voice.

Respecting autonomy thus initially requires safeguarding the ability to develop and enact autonomy, that is to say granting the other person a place in the debate, listening, revealing one's own perspective and taking the time to let the exchange evolve. At some later point, then, respecting autonomy will also entail refraining from intervening if a person has decided themselves that these actions do not harm others.

In the medical context, these presuppositions of autonomy can be translated into calls for caution and attention. For example, before following a patient's request to end life-prolonging or life-saving treatment, one ought to make sure that the patient has had time to think for themselves, the opportunity to talk to others, and, not least, that they are assured that their future existence and well-being matters. The latter entails that once a patient has reached a final decision, this decision must be regarded as authoritative. However, it also entails that the patient be assured that they will not be left alone or be perceived as a burden, should they decide to accept treatment.

Respecting autonomy thus incorporates an orientation towards well-being. It is directed at physical, psychological, and social presuppositions of autonomy. In what is to follow it will be argued that this understanding of what it means to respect autonomy is at its heart an understanding of care.

Care in Medical Ethics

The Oxford English Dictionary defines care as the "provision of what is necessary for the health, welfare, maintenance, and protection of someone or something" (Oxford Living Dictionaries 2016). Care ethicists Tronto and Fischer characterise care in the same vein as "a species of activity that includes everything we do to maintain, contain, and repair our 'world' so that we can live in it as well as possible" (Fisher and Tronto 1990, p. 40). Today's standard medical ethics approach, as introduced by American scholars Beauchamp and Childress, refers to the principles of autonomy, beneficence, non-maleficence and justice. As mentioned, care is prominent in the principles of both beneficence and non-maleficence. Beneficence calls on physicians to offer and apply only those therapies that promise to improve the patient's well-being. Non-maleficence additionally demands that medical interventions ought to have as few side effects as possible. These two principles are thus oriented towards patient well-being and contend that well-being ought to be preserved or restored, not compromised. In other words, these principles describe what care amounts to and demands.

Now, from a standard medical ethics interpretation, basing medical ethics solely on care runs the risk of justifying paternalistic attitudes and behaviour. If well-being in medicine is defined in terms of disease and illness, the experts on questions of patient well-being are the members of the healthcare team, since it is the healthcare professionals who are trained to diagnose and treat a disease and professionally care for the patient accordingly. In this scenario, it appears that healthcare team members can determine by themselves what must count as well-being for a patient. Consequently, treating and caring for a patient appears to be an activity that can be pursued independently from what the patients wants and regards as good. Restoring health is considered good for the patient, and the healthcare team itself is in the best position to judge how to accomplish this.

As a matter of fact, however, patients at the end of life may not always want to extend therapy as far as medically possible. Patients at risk of developing a disease may not always consider a strict regimen of daily preventive routines to be worth the effort. Other patients may reject specific medical interventions for religious reasons. That is to say, what constitutes well-being for an individual patient depends on how she or he values health, disease, preventive efforts, and quality of life. Stressing autonomy in medical ethics helps to incorporate this fact into healthcare practice. Following this reasoning, autonomy can be introduced as a counterbalance to care in order to push back the ethically dubious paternalistic tendencies of a solely care-based ethics.

The Care Dilemma

Nonetheless, this strategy for dealing with the supposed paternalistic tendencies of a care-based approach to medical ethics leads into a specific variation of the dilemma developed above. If one sees autonomy as prevailing over care, it becomes unclear why autonomy should be restricted to rejecting medical interventions. As long as patient preferences do not harm others, why should theses preferences not be justified? From the point of view of the autonomy principle, there can be no meaningful debate about the patient's preferences, neither based on supposedly inter-individually valid evaluations of health states, nor based on any other supposedly inter-individually valid reasons. If, however, one gives precedence to care, it must appear irrational, for example, to accept a patient's request not to undergo treatment when successful medical therapy is still possible. If the patient makes recourse to his own well-being, health care team members will be entitled to correct him or her, since defining well-being is, qua the hypothesis, part of their expertise.

What is needed in order to resolve the dilemma is an understanding of care that allows for reason-based debate about patient needs and preferences, without shifting the expertise on what is good for the patient completely into, in this case, the realm of medical and healthcare expert knowledge. Again, the hermeneutic understanding of autonomy is a viable option for resolving this dilemma. Approaching this concept from the perspective of care allows one to focus on the concept's ethical content.

Following Ricoeur, it is possible to understand autonomy as an internal dialogical process in which reasons and points of view on the good life are taken up and tested, thereby forming one's own voice. Engaging with and forming one's own will is thus inseparable from taking other perspectives into account. In his further reflection, Ricoeur equates this relation of self and other with the basic evaluational attitude of esteeming oneself and esteeming others. Indeed, one of Ricoeur's main aims is to show how being concerned with one's own will is inextricably intertwined with being concerned with the autonomy of others. When one is concerned with one's own good life, one esteems this life, and one does so also from the point of view of others. Conversely, if one cannot esteem oneself from the point of view of others and is not esteemed by others, one will not be able to esteem oneself (Ricoeur 1992, pp. 192–194). This is the reason why supporting autonomous will-formation can actually be regarded as a valuable aim from the point of view of an autonomous will. Esteeming oneself in autonomous will-formation is intimately linked to being esteemed by others and esteeming others, and ascribing to them the same abilities that one ascribes to oneself as an actor: "This exchange authorizes us to say that I cannot myself have self-esteem unless I esteem others *as* myself. 'As myself' means that you too are capable of starting something in the world, of acting for a reason, of hierarchizing your priorities, of evaluating the ends of your actions, and, having done this, of holding yourself in esteem as I hold myself in esteem" (Ricoeur 1992, p. 193). Respecting the autonomy of another thus leads to supporting the social and physical presuppositions of this kind of internal dialogue. This turn does not rest on an ethical demand that is external to what one values in autonomy. Instead, it develops within the autonomy stance itself, since autonomy presupposes esteeming others as one esteems oneself. These presuppositions can be regarded as constituting basic human needs that must be present in order to allow for autonomous will-formation.

A hermeneutic conception of care thus resolves the care dilemma by calling for attention to needs. However, these needs cannot be defined independent of the preferences of the other. First, there are physical and social needs that must be fulfilled in order to enable autonomous will-formation in general. Second, preferences might conflict with one another or with some of those very needs. Such preferences may appear puzzling from the point of view of hermeneutic care, or any understanding of care indeed, but since the aim of hermeneutic care is to enable and sustain autonomy, these preferences will have to be respected as long as due care has been taken to ensure that these preferences are not the premature results of unfulfilled social or physical needs. Care responds to needs, hermeneutic care responds to needs which enable and sustain autonomy. This specification prevents hermeneutic care from turning into paternalistic neglect of patient autonomy.

According to this account of care, caring for a patient is, first of all, caring for individual well-being insofar as it can be regarded to be a prerequisite of the ability to form a will. Health, for example, can be understood as a prerequisite of this kind. Nonetheless, humans have a capacity to individually reflect upon these prerequisites, to reject, transform, or prioritise them. Some may think there are reasons to strive for super-human powers and medical enhancements of their physical abilities. Others may regard rejecting medical treatment as the best option in their situation. Since wanting to reject a promising treatment appears to run counter to well-being, when caring for a patient one will have to learn more about why the patient prefers this option. There may be social or medical circumstances that lead to this preference which disguise an otherwise present wish to receive therapy and which one may be able to change. Caring for the patient hence involves engaging with the patient and being attentive. If one ultimately learns, however, that the kind of life that the patient will be able to have after successful treatment does not correspond to what the patient thinks of as valuable and meaningful, even if all medical and social supportive measures are in place, hermeneutic care entails refraining from attempts to override this decision, since hermeneutic care is not bound to a supposed objectively given well-being but aims at enabling and sustaining autonomous decision-making. If such a decision in a borderline case like this turns against its own prerequisites, this is disturbing. Yet ultimately, if supporting measures do not change the decision, it bears witness to what autonomous human reflection is capable of, namely neglecting itself.

In these cases, patients do not want for themselves what the health care team regards as necessary. It has been argued from the point of view of hermeneutic care that these preferences must ultimately be accepted. It is also worth noting that in cases in which the prerequisites of the autonomous will-formation of others are under threat, hermeneutic care has the resources to draw boundaries. Generally speaking, the closer an action or intention comes to threatening the very conditions of an individual to take part in a verbal or non-verbal communicative exchange of equals about reasons for actions, the more it becomes ethically dubious. At this point, Ricoeur makes use of the "golden rule". He argues that the essence of this rule is to prohibit all those actions that deprive the other of his status as an equal other in an interactive of process of determining the good. He names as examples a descending slope from influence to the betrayal of friendship and faithfulness, threat, constraint, torture and murder (Ricoeur 1992, p. 220f). All these acts are infringements on the ethical demand to treat the other just like oneself, as someone who is capable of reflecting, evaluating, and esteeming oneself and others.

Conclusion

Construing autonomy as an ethical principle along the lines of a Millean account leads to a dilemma. Relying solely on this principle makes individual decision-making look like a speechless, almost mechanistic, or at least communication free activity. However, if one introduces inter-individual reason-providing ethics accounts in addition to the autonomy principle, these accounts necessarily tend to diminish the validity of autonomy. As the dilemma stands, one must choose between contingent autonomous will on the one hand and universally prescriptive ethical demands on the other.

A hermeneutic understanding of autonomy can help us to escape this dilemma. Following Ricoeur, it can be argued that individual will-formation is a reason-guided process that necessarily involves taking the perspectives of others into account. This also holds true in those cases in which the consequences of an action or intention are exclusively borne by the actor him- or herself. Individual will-formation is directed towards the idea of a good life, the content of which cannot be determined independent of others' preferences and perspectives. Respecting autonomy, then, leads to enabling and sustaining the individual will-formation process, which is to say it leads to caring for the physical and social prerequisites of individual will-formation. Respecting autonomy, thus, comprises care. It comprises a caring attitude towards others whose autonomous will-formation is to be enabled and sustained to the greatest extent possible.

Focusing on care as prime ethical principle can, in turn, once again lead to a dilemma, since care is a reaction to needs that might appear to be objectively identifiable. This is a variation of the autonomy dilemma named above. If one gives precedence to care, it must appear irrational, for example, to accept a patient's request not to undergo treatment when successful medical therapy is still possible. If the patient makes recourse to his own well-being, health care team members will be entitled to correct him or her, since defining well-being is, qua hypothesis, part of their expertise. In contrast, if one takes recourse to a Millean account of autonomy here, it becomes unclear why autonomy should be restricted to rejecting medical interventions.

What is needed in order to resolve the dilemma is an understanding of care that allows for reason-based debate about patient needs and preferences without shifting the expertise on what is good for the patient completely into, in this case, the realm of medical and healthcare expert knowledge. Again, the hermeneutic understanding of autonomy is a viable option to resolve this dilemma. Approaching this concept from the side of care allows one to focus on the concept's care-related ethical content.

Following this line of argument, it becomes apparent that respecting the autonomy of others can be derived as an ethical demand from an understanding of individual will-formation. If one grants Ricoeur's assumption that concern for finding one's own point of view on what constitutes a good life implies esteeming oneself, then esteeming others and their points of view is a necessary part of individual will-formation, since will-formation consists of taking other perspectives into account, testing them and thereby aligning with all those who have, have had and can have a voice in this inter-individual process. Furthermore, according to this account of care, caring for a patient involves, first of all, caring for individual well-being insofar as this can be seen as a prerequisite of individual will-formation and its intersubjective, dialogical structure. These constituents of well-being may, to a large degree, be common to all humans. Health, for example, can be understood as a prerequisite of this kind. Yet if one ultimately learns that the kind of life that the patient will be able to have after successful treatment does not correspond to what the patient thinks of as valuable and meaningful, even if all medical and social supportive measures are in place, hermeneutic care entails refraining from attempts to override this decision, since hermeneutic care is not bound to a supposed objectively given state of well-being but aims at enabling and sustaining autonomous decision-making. If such a decision in a borderline case turns against its own prerequisites, this is disturbing, but ultimately, if supporting measures do not change the decision, it bears witness to what autonomous human reflection is capable of, namely neglecting itself.

Notes

1. Nicholas Agar introduced this term in Agar (2004).
2. The locus classicus of this criticism is to be found in the writings of Hegel (Hegel 1977, p. 256).
3. Most famously, Onora O'Neill has supplied a defence of a Kantian concept of autonomy in ethics and bioethics especially (O'Neill 2002).
4. Ricoeur makes use of the Aristotelian concept of phronesis to make this point (Ricoeur 1992, p. 177). He stresses that living up to this ethical aim requires "unending work of interpretation" (Ricoeur 1992, p. 179).
5. Ricoeur touches on this issue when he writes: "What we are summoned to think here is the idea of a higher finality which would never cease to be internal to human action" (Ricoeur 1992, p. 179).

References

Agar, N. (2004). *Liberal Eugenics. In Defence of Human Enhancement*. Oxford: Blackwell.

Beauchamp, T. L., & Childress, J. F. (2013). *Principles of Biomedical Ethics*. Oxford: Oxford University Press.

Fisher, B., & Tronto, J. (1990). Toward a Feminist Theory of Caring. In E. K. Abel & M. K. Nelson (Eds.), *Circles of Care. Work and Identity in Women's Lives*. Albany: State University of New York Press.

Greely, H., Campbell, P., Sahakian, B., Harris, J., Kessler, R., Gazzaniga, M., & Farah, M. J. (2008). Towards Responsible Use of Cognitive-Enhancing Drugs by the Healthy. *Nature, 456*, 702–705.

Hegel, G. W. F. (1977). *Phenomenology of Spirit* (A. V. Miller, Trans.). Oxford: Oxford University Press.

Kant, I. (1996). Groundwork of the Metaphysics of Morals. In Kant, I., *Practical Philosophy* (M. J. Gregor, Ed. & Trans.). Cambridge: Cambridge University Press.

Mill, J. S. (1869). *On Liberty*. London: Longman, Roberts & Green.

O'Neill, O. (2002). *Autonomy and Trust in Bioethics*. Cambridge: Cambridge University Press.

Oxford Living Dictionaries. (2016, December 16). English. Entry "care (noun)". Retrieved from https://en.oxforddictionaries.com/definition/care

Ricoeur, P. (1992). *Oneself as Another*. Chicago: The University of Chicago Press.

Open Access This chapter is licensed under the terms of the Creative Commons Attribution 4.0 International License (http://creativecommons.org/licenses/by/4.0/), which permits use, sharing, adaptation, distribution and reproduction in any medium or format, as long as you give appropriate credit to the original author(s) and the source, provide a link to the Creative Commons license and indicate if changes were made.

The images or other third party material in this chapter are included in the chapter's Creative Commons license, unless indicated otherwise in a credit line to the material. If material is not included in the chapter's Creative Commons license and your intended use is not permitted by statutory regulation or exceeds the permitted use, you will need to obtain permission directly from the copyright holder.

Caring Relationships: Commercial Surrogacy and the Ethical Relevance of the Other

Franziska Krause

Surrogacy and Ethics

Today commercial surrogacy is a "global baby business" (Donchin 2010, p. 323) valued at between US $500 million and US $2.0 billion in India alone (Knoche 2014). This boom in international surrogacy can be ascribed to the possibilities opened up by assisted reproductive technologies (ARTs) such as in vitro fertilisation (IVF) as well as affordable travel opportunities in the age of globalisation. Hence starting a family is no longer exclusively a question of intimacy and individual choice between two people, nor is it a question of having a vast amount of money. Surrogacy has become an attractive alternative for many couples (Robinson 2006) either when reasons of infertility or sexual orientation make a "natural" pregnancy impossible or when a woman is unwilling to carry a pregnancy. Although surrogacy is forbidden in many countries (e.g. Germany), some countries (e.g. the UK) permit altruistic surrogacy

F. Krause (✉)
Department of Medical Ethics and the History of Medicine, University of Freiburg, Freiburg, Germany

© The Author(s) 2018
F. Krause, J. Boldt (eds.), *Care in Healthcare*,
https://doi.org/10.1007/978-3-319-61291-1_6

and in others (e.g. India) surrogacy is actually a well-established form of medical tourism. Evidence suggests that the medical tourism industry will grow in the coming years, as for example, the surrogacy prices in India are five times lower than in some US states. Accordingly, Arlie Russell Hochschild describes commercial surrogacy as "the ultimate encounter between the market and intimate life" (Hochschild 2012, p. 178), where difficult questions about hiring others to perform personal acts arise. The practice of surrogacy is a sphere of life in which economic considerations, medical technologies and international regulations are indissolubly entwined. Because of its complexity, the practice of surrogacy makes ethical evaluation difficult.

Before presenting some ethical considerations concerning the practice of surrogacy, a short remark on terminology is required. In general, two kinds of surrogacy can be distinguished: In a traditional arrangement, a surrogate mother contributes her ovum and is genetically related to the child. Gestational surrogacy, in contrast, means that the surrogate carries a child that is not genetically related to her, but to the commissioning parents or a third party that donates the ovum and/or the sperm. This distinction is of empirical importance insofar as most surrogacy arrangements today are gestational and most "dramatic surrogacy failures" (Shapiro 2014, p. 1355), such as the *Baby M* case,[1] can be traced back to traditional surrogacy. Cases in which the surrogate mother is also genetically related to the child present a problem for the courts in particular, in that not only the legitimacy of surrogacy contracts has been called into question, but the issue has also been raised of whose right to the child is greater: the genetic and biological mother, or the genetic father and his wife, the social mother.

However, gestational surrogacy without apparent conflicts, which is relatively routine today, is not suited to serve as a starting point for a moral evaluation of the practice of surrogacy, and it is even less suited to present a moral argument to legitimise surrogacy. It can merely serve to emphasise different manifestations of problems within the *practice* of surrogacy. And even though ethical questions, such as the role of embodiment and genetic ties, are of greater importance in traditional than in gestational arrangements, I will show that both arrangements can share the problem of disconnected relationships. In this chapter, I consider relationships to be an essential component for taking on responsibility. But this also requires that a relationship is recognised as such—a requirement which, above all in commercial surrogacy arrangements, is rarely fulfilled.

In addition to the distinction between gestational and traditional surrogacy, some authors draw a distinction between commercial and altruistic surrogacy in order to underline that the motivation for becoming a surrogate mother is central to the moral status of surrogacy itself. Many ethicists interpreting surrogacy as an arrangement of exploitation[2] and commodification[3] refer to the vulnerable socio-economic background of most surrogates and suspect them of having become a surrogate solely out of financial motivation. Because of this financial incentive, the surrogate's decision cannot be declared as autonomous (which is the basis for "right" actions) but as heteronomous, that is guided by external motivations. Indeed, the financial incentive for women in the "global south" to enter into a surrogacy arrangement is extremely high. A woman who works as a surrogate can assure the livelihood of her family for five years; furthermore, she is able to offer her own children a better future by sending them to school (Karandikar et al. 2014; Panitch 2013). Besides the status of financial compensation in surrogacy arrangements, other conditions are problematic as well. The educational level of the surrogates is low, which often prevents them from understanding the contract conditions, the medical risks[4] and the procedures they will have to undergo. There is a danger that the surrogates will make their decision under non-ideal circumstances and agree to give birth to a child that is not theirs in absence of the conditions for informed consent. Furthermore, their lack of education also diminishes their opportunities for other jobs. As a consequence, surrogacy often appears to be the only option these women have (Pande 2010). On the basis of the socio-economic conditions of most surrogates in the global south, surrogacy can be interpreted in one sense as providing the wrong financial incentive to do something one would not otherwise do or, alternatively, as a realistic chance for the surrogates and their families to live a better (autonomous) life (Fabre 2006; Macklin 1990).

From a libertarian standpoint, none of these socio-economic conditions constitutes a reason to forbid surrogacy per se. A prohibition is considered to be a restriction of the freedom of women rather than a protection against exploitation. Prohibiting surrogacy would diminish women's autonomy and freedom of choice unjustifiably. Richard Arneson describes the libertarian position as follows:

> No matter how restricted one's life options, the idea that the narrow range of one's options unacceptably constrains one's choice is not a reason to limit further one's range of choice. (Arneson 1992, p. 158)

In line with this opinion, Cécile Fabre argues that even though women in India often opt for surrogacy under non-ideal conditions (which should be improved), they live a "minimally flourishing life" (Fabre 2006, p. 187), which ensures that they can decide freely and in accordance with life plans. Any notion of further concerns, for example the emotional distress of being pregnant and giving birth to a child for another couple, is something that has to be taken seriously, but is no reason to deny people the possibility of choosing surrogacy (Fabre 2006, p. 199). Indeed, Fabre even allows surrogates to keep the child because of emotional ties; however, from her standpoint this is a question of "valid, but voidable contracts" (Fabre 2006, pp. 186–218). The eventuality of emotional bonding does not constitute a reason to doubt the correctness of the surrogacy contracts themselves. Even though some studies show empirical evidence that bonding between mother and child during pregnancy does not necessarily occur (Robbins and Eaves 2013), the question remains whether the *possibility* of bonding and the consequential potential harm to the surrogate is a real challenge for the practice of surrogacy. These doubts are dismissed by Fabre: "we cannot and will not ever be able to live in a risk-free society, particularly one free of the emotional risks attendant on parenthood. Nor, in fact, should we aspire to do so" (Fabre 2006, p. 218).

Other authors who also do not condemn contract surrogacy in general, but are rather concerned with gender inequality in the practice of surrogacy, mention the need to take care of "the most economically and emotionally vulnerable party in any such arrangement" (Satz 2010, p. 132), that is the surrogate, and thus demand an improvement in the conditions of surrogates in the global south. This may include, for instance, making third-party brokerage of pregnancy contracts illegal, giving women the right to terminate the pregnancy against the will of the commissioning parents or making educational and occupational programmes available to Indian women. As a result of such measures, fewer Indian women would "choose" to become gestational surrogates (Satz 2010; Schanbacher 2014). Leaving aside the feasibility of the implementation of these requirements as part of the practice of surrogacy, the question as to the moral and social consequences of even an ideal practice of surrogacy still remains.

Already in the 1980s, the feminist philosopher Susan Sherwin claimed that it was a task for medical ethics to analyse ARTs in the context of control over reproduction. For her it is obvious that the increased use of ARTs, such as IVF, and the possibility of surrogate pregnancy imply a decrease in women's control over their reproduction—especially for the surrogates.[5] We must look not just to broad social policy, but also to the details of relationships to delineate the social attitudes and patterns that are at risk of being undermined (Sherwin 1989). The analysis must not be restricted to the individual and its situation nor to dyadic and personal relationships, but rather it must consider the relationships of all parties involved. Recently the care-ethicist Stephanie Collins wrote that, based on the inherent value relationships have for people, "relationships ought to be (a) treated as moral paradigms, (b) valued, preserved, or promoted (as appropriate to the circumstances at hand), and (c) acknowledged as giving rise to weighty duties" (Collins 2015, p. 47). This leads to the crucial question of what the moral foundation of relationships is and why relationships are important to individuals.

Levinas and Ethics

A philosopher for whom the relationship with another person is central for morality and for ethics is Emmanuel Levinas. Based on a phenomenological methodology presented with Jewish-theological thinking and terms, he describes ethics as an intersubjective relation beyond the need of any consciousness, knowledge or reflective ability. Levinas' ethics can be read in the tradition of phenomenology. He describes the phenomenon of life by posing the question of what something means for us as human beings. In an ongoing process of perceiving and interacting with the world, the self finds what it means to be ethical. For Levinas, ethics is the first and most important discipline of philosophy. However, his understanding of ethics differs from traditional ethical theories. It is neither based on a Kantian idea of self-legislation, nor the calculation of happiness, such as in utilitarianism, nor the cultivation of virtues. Instead it is best understood as a proto-ethics. This means that it focuses on the question of what it takes to understand ethics and why people should be moral at all. The idea of weighing different ethical principles is not relevant to Levinas, insofar as he describes an ethics which initially only addresses the relationship of the self to the Other and what it means for the self to carry responsibility for the Other. Questions involving the needs of many people, for example concerning justice, are of subordinate interest to Levinas. Being-with-one-another is an ontological dimension of a person and not just a social fact without any impact on the individual. This is why the foundation of Levinas' approach centres on the face-to-face encounter of the self and the so-called Other. The fact that Levinas presents the Other as fundamentally dissimilar, that is not merely as another self (the Not-I) or someone who displays similar characteristics, opens up the possibility, according to Levinas, to avoid reducing the Other in the self to a certain facet or a particular notion of the Other.[6]

Levinas and the Ethics of Care: The Mother–Child Relationship

Even though Levinas never uses the word "care" to describe the relationship between the self and the Other, the ethics of care and Levinas have a lot in common. Both take the mother–child relationship as a paradigm of their anthropological analysis. Although the phenomenology of natality is described as having all the aspects of a maternal body, the concept of the mother is not exclusive to women but rather independent of any category of sex. The relationship between mother and child serves as a paradigm for the fundamental vulnerability and dependency of the self. Without the mother, a child would not have been born and could not be part of this world. Life thus begins with dependency and with an asymmetry of power, and both these characteristics of life require the care of another person. Being in a relationship with someone is therefore the first condition for being in the world. An ethics which emerges from such an image of human contingency and dependency represents an alternative to the model that regards people as "self-interested strangers" (Held 2006, p. 77) who simply enter into a contract with each other. It highlights responsibilities which exceed contractual models of reciprocity.

Furthermore, the mother–child relationship sheds light on the special characteristic of ethical relations: In the eyes of the mother, her child is special. Because of the fact of natality—which plays a crucial role both in the ethics of care and for Levinas—the concept of humankind starts with an emphasis on the particularity of every person and every situation. Just as the child is special to the mother, all people are of importance to someone. They are unique and irreplaceable in their meaning to someone else.

Finally, both ethics underline the importance of the attitude of being responsive to the Other and the world. Being responsive is not something one can really choose to be. Levinas uses the image of "being held hostage" to describe the phenomenon of dependency. In pregnancy, this dependency becomes obvious. Having a baby limits the freedom of the mother—she is not supposed to drink or eat what she wants, her body changes enormously and feeling physically sick is often part of pregnancy. It is not unusual for women to wish for their "customary body" back (Staehler 2016, p. 31), that is the ability to perform everyday activities again as usual. A mother's love for her child is not affected by these constraints, however. According to Levinas, the same is true for the relationship with the Other: Being in a relationship with the Other represents a challenge for the self. This relationship is not freely chosen in its conditions, but is based on unconditional responsiveness and responsibility towards the Other.

Being responsive and responding to the needs of someone else are thus central to both Levinas and the ethics of care. While Levinas primarily foregrounds the needs of the Other, an ethics of care also asks to what extent the self can fulfil the needs of the Other. According to the well-known definition by the care-ethicist Joan Tronto (Tronto 1993, 2013), care is best understood as attitude and as practice. While this differentiation can be made methodologically, in daily life the phases of care often occur (or at least should occur) all at once. "Caring about" and "taking care of" are descriptions of the attitude of the care-giver while "care-giving" and "care-receiving" touch on the practice of care. "To care" is about assessing a need (attentiveness), realising that one has the capabilities to help the other (responsibility), coming in contact with the object of care (competence) and expecting a response from the care-receiver (responsiveness) (Tronto 2013, pp. 34–35). Although the Other obviously plays a crucial role in the process of caring, almost all discussions about caring start from the perspective of the care-giver and not the care-receiver, as Tronto states (Tronto 2013, p. 150). This is the point where Levinas can offer important insights to supplement the ethics of care, because he builds his concept of relationships on the role of the care-receiver, the so-called Other. While the ethics of care can create awareness of how care practices should ideally proceed and the social, economic and political conditions necessary to facilitate this, Levinas lays the foundation for understanding why the Other approaches us and why we have to take responsibility for them. Levinas locates answers to the "why" of care in the Other, and not in the self.

Levinas' Concept of Responsibility

Levinas' starting point for ethics is the Other. The Other contains a transcendent part, a part which exceeds all experiences in the real world. Alterity—the being totally different than the self and different than any other object of experience—is addressing the self. It is challenging the self to give an adequate answer, because the self desires to understand the Other, but also lacks the capacity to fulfil this aspiration.

The relation to the Other is ethical, which for Levinas means that the self has to overcome traditional categories of thinking and acting, and that infinite responsibility for the Other is the mode of their relationship. This responsibility cannot be delegated, even if someone else can respond in a given situation. However, this should not be understood as an actual responsibility but rather as something pre-ontological that gives rise to a motivation to act ethically and to care for the welfare of the Other. How to respond to the call of the Other and to exercise one's own responsibility is up to the self and its judgement:

> The will is free to assume this responsibility in whatever sense it likes; it is not free to refuse this responsibility itself; it is not free to ignore the meaningful world into which the face of the Other has introduced it. (Levinas 1991b, pp. 218–219)

When Eva Feder Kittay says that it must first be acknowledged that who is responsible for whom is often a matter of absolute judgement and less a matter of degree (Feder Kittay 1999, p. 56), she is actually making the same point as Levinas. To meet the needs of another person is an absolute necessity and cannot be rejected, because without the Other, the self would not be obliged to give reasons for its action or even identify its own capacity to act. The question of the right reaction to the need of the Other, that is the actualisation of responsibility, is secondary. In this way, Levinas' conception of responsibility differs from what we usually think of when we talk about responsibility: The ability to act is typically understood to be a necessary condition for recognising and exercising responsibility. For Levinas, in contrast, being responsible for the Other is the foundation of every action. Before you act, you are already responsible.

The passivity of the self that is expressed by "being-already-in-responsibility" is why Levinas' concept of responsibility cannot be attributed to an intentional act; it is nothing the self can decide on. However, responsibility is normative, because it is necessary in order to be ethical, to be part of humanity. Thus, from Levinas' point of view, one may even say that the Other constitutes the self in its morality, because without the Other there would be no reason for being moral. Although the absolute responsibility for the Other seems to force the self into heteronomous actions, as Levinas sees it, this mode of relation constitutes an antecedent to freedom and the condition for being ethical. From this perspective, freedom is best understood as a liberation from ontological necessities, a "deliverance from Being" (Ciaramelli 1991, p. 88). The way Levinas thinks about the self also becomes clearer in this context: It is not a Hobbesian self that identifies the Other as a risk for one's own life and freedom. Instead the self is ethical and becomes a subject of good will with the appearance of the Other, because "*toward another* culminates in *for another*" (Levinas 1991a, p. 18).

Levinas even goes a step further by claiming that the relationship to the Other is of a general non-reciprocal asymmetry. The self does not expect any kind of compensation in return for its responsibility to meet the needs of the Other. Within the ethical relation, the Other and the self are so different that it is impossible to conclude that the Other also has a responsibility for the self. The attempt to draw an analogy between the self and the Other fails, because the Other is characterised by an absolute alterity,[7] a transcendent part, as Levinas calls it. This transcendent part of the Other renders the expectation of reciprocity or symmetry within the concept of responsibility impossible:

> The knot of subjectivity consists in going to the other without concerning oneself with his movement toward me. [...] I have always one response more to give, I have to answer for his very responsibility. (Levinas 1991a, p. 84)

Whereas there are no restrictions on the responsibility of the self for the Other—even the responsibility of the Other devolves upon the self—the self cannot expect the other to behave in the same manner. To be is first of all being for the Other without expecting a reward. For Levinas, seeking reciprocity refers to the sphere of economy, that is to mere contracts. Within a contract there is no need to recognise the alterity of the Other, because economic relations are based on utility and the expectation of reciprocity between equals. Mere economy epitomises the "totalisation of unique persons" (Levinas 1995, p. 54). In this sphere, there is just a numerical alterity or diversity of Others, not a kind of recognition of the alterity of the Other. In contrast, ethics is the opposite. Ethics requires relationships between unique individuals and the recognition of their alterity. As a consequence, the purpose of ethics is not a search for rules or principles, but rather a search for the right response to a concrete Other.

Levinas and the Concept of Relational Autonomy

Levinas' conception of ethics is furthermore a warning not to place a specific concept of the self at the centre of ethics. According to Levinas, a self that has been reduced to self-consciousness and self-sufficiency is untenable. This critique can be read as a provocative shift of emphasis in times where the self and its autonomy are conceptualised as acting "freely in accordance with a self-chosen plan" (Beauchamp and Childress 2009, p. 99), that is where self-reference is central. When Levinas refers to the self, he is referring to a subjectivity that exists in dialogue and not as ego. Of course, a "life of enjoyment" and independence from the Other are also part of the self. Enjoyment is not tied to an end; it is the hedonistic sensibility beyond any act of consciousness. In this sense, Levinas anticipates the critique of the absolute passivity of the self that may lead to a loss of self. However, the self of enjoyment is the self "who gives to the Other when called upon in the face-to-face relation" (Chanter 2005, p. 42). Only a self that is different from the Other can be for the Other. The aspect of enjoyment helps to emphasise this ontological and epistemological distinction between the Other and the self. In contrast, the self and the Other interact intensely on the ethical level. They do not just share the world with each other; instead, the Other is welcomed into a world of "hospitality." It is necessary to include the Other in order to be ethical, to be responsive and to perceive the necessity of acting.

> Vulnerability, exposure to outrage, to wounding, passivity more passive than all patience, passivity of the accusative form, trauma of accusation suffered by a hostage to the point of persecution, implicating the identity of the hostage who substitutes himself for the others: all this is the self, a defecting or defeat of the ego's identity. And this, pushed to the limit, is sensibility, sensibility as the subjectivity of the subject. It is a substitution for another, one in the place of another, expiation. (Levinas 1991a, p. 15)

The passivity of the ethical self is connected to the ontological vulnerability of the self, namely its susceptibility to various harms or exploitations. For Levinas, vulnerability is the basis for sensibility, for being responsive to the Other. In recent years, the discussion about vulnerability and relationality of the self also became an integral element of the discussion about "relational autonomy." Catriona Mackenzie and Natalie Stoljar characterise relational autonomy as follows:

> The focus of relational approaches is to analyse the implications of the intersubjective and social dimensions of selfhood and identity for conceptions of individual autonomy and moral and political agency. (Mackenzie and Stoljar 2000, p. 4)

They consider the exercise of individual autonomy to be embedded in historical and social features and therefore criticise, for example libertarians, for paying little attention to the background social conditions in which preferences are formed (Mackenzie 2014). Social structures and interpersonal relations are not just to be considered as a condition of causal control, instead they partly generate autonomy by affecting one's capacity to live an "autonomous" life (Dodds 2007; Oshana 2006; Westlund 2009). In other words, autonomy is constituted by the social, personal, economic and cultural embeddedness of the self and is an ongoing process that takes place in relation to others. In this sense, relationships should not be understood as intrinsically good; they also exhibit a disruptive potential—for example, when they prevent a self-determined life from being led or undermine shared values. Thus, questions such as those regarding the emancipation from oppression, the recognition of the Other and how best to structure our social practices in order to allow for autonomy are of particular importance.

These insights can help to clarify what a relational approach to the practice of surrogacy means: Relationships are an indispensable part of constituting the self, and in the context of surrogacy, this leads to a reconsideration of the importance of all kinds of relationships inherent to the practice of surrogacy as part of an ethical evaluation. To look at the practice of surrogacy as an individuals' choice (as libertarian positions do) means to refuse the complexity of such arrangements. Neither is the surrogate solipsistic in her autonomy nor is the decision of the commissioning parents independent of the social world they live in.

Levinas and Surrogacy

When Elizabeth Anderson states with regard to surrogacy that "by engaging in the transfer for children by sale, all of the parties to the surrogate contract express a set of attitudes toward children which undermine the norms of parental love" (Anderson 1990, p. 77), she seems to agree with Levinas. Contracts cannot regulate the way in which people should feel responsible for the concrete Other. Contractual arrangements suggest that a parental relationship starts when the parents-to-be bring the child back to their home country. In line with Levinas, it is possible to explain why the responsibility of the parents-to-be is not limited to the baby, but has to be extended to the surrogate. In order to form a more precise idea of the shared responsibilities and the parties involved in surrogacy arrangements, however, drawing a distinction from Levinas seems to be informative. In general, three kinds of relationship can be ascribed to surrogacy arrangements (setting aside surrogacy agencies or sperm and ovum donors).

First of all, there is the relationship between mother and child. This relationship is central for Levinas' concept of being ethical, because pregnancy exhibits the same features as being a moral agent: Not all responsibilities for the Other are freely chosen, but the experience of the good is ubiquitous. The surrogate is bodily intertwined with the baby, and she "cannot choose not to be morally responsible for the fetus while it remains in her womb. In this sense, biology is certainly destiny" (van Zyl and van Niekerk 2000, p. 407). The relationship to the baby is based on sensibility beyond any genetic ties. It is not a question of knowledge of the Other or of the level of cognitive reflection, but it is instead the corporeal experience of the Other which determines its own dimension of cognition and experience. Levinas characterises this corporeal experience as sensibility, which is present in every cognitive-reflexive experience of the self, thus:

> Sensibility—the proximity, immediacy and restlessness which signify in it—is not constituted out of some apperception putting consciousness into relation with a body. Incarnation is not a transcendental operation of a subject that is situated in the midst of the world it represents to itself; the sensible experience of the body is already and from the start incarnate. The sensible—maternity, vulnerability, apprehension—binds the node of incarnation into a plot larger than the apperception of self. (Levinas 1991a, p. 76)

The corporeal experience is much more powerful than a conscious examination of the self and the world can be. In this sense, alienation from the Other, the baby, is secondary to the immediate experience of the Other and only imaginable as a reflective and conscious act. This conscious alienation is exactly what agencies demand from the surrogates:

not to feel a deep connectedness to the baby, but rather to consider their wombs as "carriers" and themselves just as "prenatal babysitters" (Hochschild 2011, p. 24). From a phenomenological perspective, however, the body cannot be viewed exclusively as an object of ownership and control, but is rather a gateway to the world for the purpose of sensibility, which has proven itself independent of cognitive reflection. The concept of the "lived body," which is greatly emphasised in phenomenology for its experience of the self (Carel 2011; Folkmarson Käll and Zeiler 2014), is knowingly manipulated and denied by agencies in the practice of surrogacy. Here mothers are prevented from bonding with the child during pregnancy, as this could potentially lead to the refusal to handover the child to the contracted parents and consequently result in a breach of contract—such as in the case of Baby M.

A second kind of relationship takes place between the parents-to-be and the baby that can be described in Levinas words as fatherhood. The main characteristic of fatherhood is not corporeity, but rather the uniqueness a father attributes to his child:

> The son is a unique son. Not by number; each son of the father is the unique son, the chosen son. The love of the father for the son accomplishes the sole relation. (Levinas 1991b, p. 279)

Whereas the image of the Other in the self plays a role in motherhood, the recognition of the Other in its Otherness figures in fatherhood. Therefore, it is a not a matter of defining the role of genetic paternity and the responsibility associated with it, but instead a matter of Finding-Yourself-in-the-Other without being the Other. Responsibility and attachment are thus seen as a process of recognition. The commissioning parents have a similar relation to the child—regardless of whether they are genetically related to the child or not. They are looking for their unique child and want to assume responsibility for the child's whole life. However, as some cases in the practice of surrogacy show, this responsibility is a fragile construct.[8] Unconditional love can be compromised and depreciated by the existence of a contract that seems to regulate the needs and responsibilities inherent in surrogacy arrangements (Kuhlmann 1998). Surrogacy contracts imply the possibility of control over the purchased product, yet fail to recognise that in the case of a child, the contract does not concern goods, but instead a person who is vulnerable and non-exchangeable in their uniqueness.

The relationship between the surrogate and the parents-to-be is the third relationship of special importance in surrogacy arrangements. Little attention is paid to this topic in scientific discourse, but for this analysis it is crucial to show that the surrogate and the commissioning parents are not just contract partners, but also interrelated in an ethical manner. Levinas' concept of "the third" offers an interesting insight for the analysis of this special relationship, as it shatters the private relationship between the self and the Other and introduces a different, although still ethical, quality. As Stéphane Mosès points out, the third is different from the Other in the sense of proximity, quantity and its selection: The third is further afar than the Other, it is numerous instead of unique, and it is the only one in an ethical relationship that is freely chosen (Mosès 1993). The surrogates meet the criteria: they are usually miles away from the commissioning parents, it does not matter to them exactly which surrogate carries their child to term, and it is they who choose to enter a surrogacy arrangement and involve a third party in their family planning.

However, for Levinas, the third does not need to be conceived as a visible empirical human being. Instead, it is best interpreted as reminder that other people who are not part of a personal relationship and differ from the self in terms of ethnicity, sex, status or religion must be considered as well. The third interferes with the relationship of the self and the Other and thereby challenges the privileged position of the Other. Thus, it opens up the frontiers of thinking. The relationship to the third is not personal anymore, but refers to the sphere of justice and equality.[9] Therefore, the third is also allied with institutions and universal laws instead of the particularity and context-sensitivity that is part of personal relationships. Levinas comments on the difference between the Other and the third as being a difference in thinking:

> [...] what seems to me very important, is that there are not only two of us in the world. But I think that everything begins as if we were only two. It is important to recognize that the idea of justice always supposes that there is a third. But, initially, in principle, I am concerned about justice because the other has a face. (Levinas et al. 2005, p. 170)

It is notable that Levinas recognises that we need institutions and relationships of reciprocity and equality. However, this cannot mean that the social and the political sphere—what he calls "justice"—render the face of the Other irrelevant. Quite the contrary: The presence of the Other must not be replaced by institutional structures. Responsibility is always present as if there were a concrete Other with specific needs. For the practice of surrogacy this means that even though the surrogate is not part of a personal relationship, she is nevertheless part of a personal responsibility, and her needs must be met. In the current situation it is easy for the commissioning parents to shake off their responsibilities by referring to contracts with the agencies or to the fulfilment of governmental instructions. This is a development that Levinas criticises in his work: Institutionalisation, that is the mere application of rules, principles and laws, allows people to forget that exercising responsibility for the Other is valuable in order to do justice. Alternatively, one may say that ethics needs forms of institutionalisation but this set of (universal) rules must serve ethics. And ethics is capable of forming a better society only if people accept their personal responsibilities.

Conclusion

The discourse about the global practice of surrogacy often focuses on the question of the exploitation of surrogates or the increasing commercialisation of our lives. The point of view presented in this paper does not dispute such arguments, nor does it offer new concepts for dealing with the practice of surrogacy. It rather demonstrates a shift in perspective in order to provide a broader overview about the risks of surrogacy arrangements, with a special emphasis on the responsibilities in relationships that are often subverted in commercial surrogacy. Despite its importance, the role of the commissioning parents in particular receives little attention in ethical discourse. This is surprising insofar as without the parents-to-be, the demand for surrogacy arrangements would not exist, and the ethical debate would appear more or less redundant. New forms of relationships are born in the context of ARTs—such as the one between surrogates and the commissioning parents—but the allocation of responsibilities remains unclear. This gap can be filled by Levinas' arguments about relationships of responsibility. First of all, he shows that relationships constitute the self as moral or ethical. Being dependent on others is not a form of oppression but rather the condition for understanding the capacity of accepting responsibility. Furthermore, relationships of responsibility are not restricted to dyadic and personalities, because, particularly today, the parties involved in relationships are numerous, and people are indissolubly bound to each other as a result of global interdependence. Although relationships exhibit different modes of actualising responsibilities, this does not diminish the responsibility per se. In addition to this phenomenological description of relationships, Levinas can be read as a critical voice on the idea that international regulation is the main issue in the context of surrogacy. From Levinas' standpoint, such an argument obfuscates the real search for justice, which must be located in the self and its responsibility. Being ethical is nothing definitive, but rather an individual's endless search for an adequate way of being-for-the-Other. All these deliberations coincide with a reading in terms of the ethics of care insofar as revealing the need to take on responsibility can be read as a first step in overcoming the "crises of care" (Parks 2010)—as Jennifer Parks characterises the practice of surrogacy.

Notes

1. Elizabeth and William Stern entered into a surrogacy contract with Marybeth Whitehead. In 1986 Whitehead gave birth to a girl, Baby M, but was unable or unwilling to surrender the child to the Sterns. As William Stern was the legal father of the child, having provided the sperm, and Marybeth Whitehead the biological and genetic mother of the child, a court battle over custody extended over several years.
2. For the different facets of exploitation in surrogacy arrangements, see Wertheimer (1992).
3. Commodification is the idea that the norms of the market are appropriate for regulating its production, exchange and enjoyment. Critics regard this as a fatal economisation of the social. cf.: Anderson (1990).
4. One of the main medical risks of surrogacy is the caesarean delivery that is often forced onto the surrogate in order to accommodate the paying couple. See: Knoche (2014).
5. Of course, it can also be argued that the infertile woman who seeks a child is a potential victim of power relations in our society as she is *expected* to

use all available reproductive technologies to fulfil her dream of her own child.

6. Even Martin Heidegger, with whose philosophy Levinas was well acquainted, characterises the ontological structure of the human being (Dasein) as relationality, the "being-with" (Mitsein), in his book *Being and Time*. The Other contributes significantly to the development of the self. On Heidegger's relationality, Freeman writes: "Human beings are constituted by their relational, ontological structure of Mitsein, which is neither added on to Dasein as an afterthought nor derivative of it" (Freeman 2011, p. 368). Levinas goes far beyond considering being-with (Mitsein) as a phenomenon in which the self is found. Levinas characterises the relationship to the Other as an ethical relationship which challenges the self in itself and in which the self is continuously searching for the appropriate response to the needs of the Other. While for Levinas, the relationship to the Other is essential for selfhood, Heidegger concentrated on the significance of the world and the Other for the Dasein of the self in its mineness (Jemeinigkeit).
7. This concept is criticised by Derrida: "The Other cannot be absolved of a relation to an ego from which it is other; it cannot be absolutely Other." Compare: Bernasconi (2000).
8. For example, in the case of Baby Manji, the Japanese commissioning parents divorced during the pregnancy and rejected their child. Ultimately, the grandmother adopted Baby Manji—otherwise the Baby would have remained parentless and stateless.
9. Most authors describe the third as Levinas' concept of the political sphere. See: Bedorf (2003); Caygill (2002); Delhom (2000); Simmons (1999).

References

Anderson, E. S. (1990). Is Women's Labor a Commodity? *Philosophy & Public Affairs, 19*(1s), 71–92.

Arneson, R. J. (1992). Commodification and Commercial Surrogacy. *Philosophy & Public Affairs, 21*(2s), 132–164.

Beauchamp, T. L. and Childress, J. F. (2009). *Principles of Biomedical Ethics*. Oxford: Oxford University Press.

Bedorf, T. (2003). *Dimensionen des Dritten. Sozialphilosophische Modelle zwischen Ethischem und Politischem*. München: Wilhelm Fink Verlag.

Bernasconi, R. (2000). The Alterity of the Stranger and the Experience of the Alien. In J. Bloechl (Ed.), *The Face of the Other and the Trace of God. Essays on*

the Philosophy of Emmanuel Levinas (pp. 62–89). New York: Fordham University Press.
Carel, H. (2011). Phenomenology and Its Application in Medicine. *Theoretical Medicine and Bioethics, 32*(1s), 33–46.
Caygill, H. (2002). *Levinas and the Political.* London: Routledge.
Chanter, T. (2005). Feminism and the Other. In R. Bernasconi & D. Wood (Eds.), *The Provocation of Levinas. Rethinking the Other* (pp. 32–56). London: Routledge.
Ciaramelli, F. (1991). Levinas's Ethical Discourse Between Individuation and Universality. In R. Bernasconi & S. Critchley (Eds.), *Re-reading Levinas* (pp. 83–105). Bloomington: Indiana University Press.
Collins, S. (2015). *The Core of Care Ethics.* New York: Palgrave Macmillan.
Delhom, P. (2000). *Der Dritte. Lévinas' Philosophie zwischen Verantwortung und Gerechtigkeit.* München: Wilhelm Fink.
Dodds, S. (2007). Depending on Care. Recognition of Vulnerability and the Social Contribution of Care Provision. *Bioethics, 21*(9s), 500–510.
Donchin, A. (2010). Reproductive Tourism and the Quest for Global Gender Justice. *Bioethics, 24*(7s), 323–332.
Fabre, C. (2006). *Whose Body Is It Anyway? Justice and the Integrity of the Person.* Oxford: Clarendon Press.
Feder Kittay, E. (1999). *Love's Labor. Essays on Women, Equality and Dependency.* New York: Routledge.
Folkmarson Käll, L., & Zeiler, K. (2014). Bodily Relational Autonomy. *Journal of Consciousness Studies, 21*(9s), 100–120.
Freeman, L. (2011). Reconsidering Relational Autonomy. A Feminist Approach to Selfhood and the Other in the Thinking of Martin Heidegger. *Inquiry, 54*(4s), 361–383.
Held, V. (2006). *The Ethics of Care. Personal, Political and Global.* Oxford: Oxford University Press.
Hochschild, A. (2011). Emotional Life on the Market Frontier. *Annual Review of Sociology, 37*, 21–33.
Hochschild, A. R. (2012). *The Outsourced Self.* New York: Henry Holt.
Karandikar, S., Gezinski, L. B., Carter, J. R., & Kaloga, M. (2014). Economic Necessity or Noble Cause? A Qualitative Study Exploring Motivations for Gestational Surrogacy in Gujarat, India. *Affilia, 29*(2s), 224–236.
Knoche, J. W. (2014). Health Concerns and Ethical Considerations Regarding International Surrogacy. *International Journal of Gynecology and Obstetrics, 126*(2s), 183–186.
Kuhlmann, A. (1998). Reproduktive Autonomie? Zur Denaturierung der menschlichen Fortpflanzung. *Deutsche Zeitschrift für Philosophie, 46*(6s), 917–933.

Levinas, E. (1991a). *Otherwise than Being or Beyond Essence*. Dordrecht: Kluwer Academic Publishers.

Levinas, E. (1991b). *Totality and Infinity. An Essay on Exteriority*. Dordrecht: Kluwer Academic Publishers.

Levinas, E. (1995). *Zwischen uns. Versuche über das Denken und den Anderen*. München: Hanser.

Levinas, E., Wright, T., Hughes, P. and Ainley, A. (2005). The Paradox of Morality. An Interview with Emmanuel Levinas. In R. Bernasconi and D. Wood (Eds.), *The Provocation of Levinas. Rethinking the Other* (pp. 168–180). London: Routledge.

Mackenzie, C. (2014). The Importance of Relational Autonomy and Capabilities for an Ethics of Vulnerability. In C. Mackenzie, W. Rogers and S. Dodds (Eds.), *Vulnerability. New Essays in Ethics and Feminist Philosophy* (pp. 33–59). New York: Oxford University Press.

Mackenzie, C. and Stoljar, N. (2000). Introduction. Autonomy Refigured. In C. Mackenzie and N. Stoljar (Eds.), *Relational Autonomy. Feminist Perspectives on Autonomy, Agency, and the Social Self* (pp. 3–31). New York: Oxford University Press.

Macklin, R. (1990). Is There Anything Wrong with Surrogate Motherhood? In L. Gostin (Ed.), *Surrogate Motherhood* (pp. 136–149). Bloomington: Indiana University Press.

Mosès, S. (1993). Gerechtigkeit und Gemeinschaft bei Emmanuel Lévinas. In M. Brumlik and H. Brunkhorst (Eds.), *Gemeinschaft und Gerechtigkeit* (pp. 364–384). Frankfurt a.M.: Fischer.

Oshana, M. (2006). *Personal Autonomy in Society*. Aldershot: Ashgate.

Pande, A. (2010). "At Least I Am Not Sleeping with Anyone". Resisting the Stigma of Commercial Surrogacy in India. *Feminist Studies, 36*(2s), 292–312.

Panitch, V. (2013). Surrogate Tourism and Reproductive Rights. *Hypatia, 28*(2s), 274–289.

Parks, J. A. (2010). Care Ethics and the Global Practice of Commercial Surrogacy. *Bioethics, 24*(7s), 333–340.

Robbins, A., & Eaves, A. (2013). Meet the Baby Carriers. Available at: http://www.washingtonian.com/articles/work-education/meet-the-baby-carriers/. Accessed 28 Aug 2013.

Robinson, F. (2006). Ethical Globalization? States, Corporations, and the Ethics of Care. In M. Hamington and D. C. Miller (Eds.), *Socializing Care* (pp. 163–181). Lanham: Rowman & Littlefield Publishers.

Satz, D. (2010). *Why Some Things Should Not Be for Sale*. Oxford: Oxford University Press.

Schanbacher, K. (2014). India's Gestational Surrogacy Market. An Exploitation of Poor, Uneducated Women. *Hastings Women's Law Journal, 25*(2s), 201–220.

Shapiro, J. (2014). For a Feminist Considering Surrogacy, Is Compensation Really the Key Question? *Washington Law Review, 89*, 1345–1373.

Sherwin, S. (1989). Feminist and Medical Ethics. Two Different Approaches to Contextual Ethics. *Hypatia, 4*(2s), 57–72.

Simmons, W. (1999). The Third. Levinas' Theoretical Move from An-archical Ethics to the Realm of Justice and Politics. *Philosophy & Social Criticism, 25*(6s), 83–104.

Staehler, T. (2016). Vom Berührtwerden. Schwangerschaft als paradoxes Paradigma. In H. Landweer and I. Marcinski (Eds.), *Dem Erleben auf der Spur. Feminismus und die Philosophie des Leibes* (pp. 27–43). Bielefeld: transcript.

Tronto, J. C. (1993). *Moral Boundaries. A Political Argument for an Ethics of Care*. New York: Routledge.

Tronto, J. C. (2013). *Caring Democracy. Markets, Equality and Justice*. New York: New York University Press.

van Zyl, L. and van Niekerk, A. (2000). Interpretations, Perspectives and Intentions in Surrogate Motherhood. *Journal of Medical Ethics, 26*, 404–409.

Wertheimer, A. (1992). Two Questions About Surrogacy and Exploitation. *Philosophy & Public Affairs, 21*(3s), 211–239.

Westlund, A. C. (2009). Rethinking Relational Autonomy. *Hypatia, 24*(4s), 26–49.

Open Access This chapter is licensed under the terms of the Creative Commons Attribution 4.0 International License (http://creativecommons.org/licenses/by/4.0/), which permits use, sharing, adaptation, distribution and reproduction in any medium or format, as long as you give appropriate credit to the original author(s) and the source, provide a link to the Creative Commons license and indicate if changes were made.

The images or other third party material in this chapter are included in the chapter's Creative Commons license, unless indicated otherwise in a credit line to the material. If material is not included in the chapter's Creative Commons license and your intended use is not permitted by statutory regulation or exceeds the permitted use, you will need to obtain permission directly from the copyright holder.

Situated Care

Sociomaterial Will-Work: Aligning Daily Wanting in Dutch Dementia Care

Annelieke Driessen

'Daily Wanting' in Dementia Care

Then,[1] finally, Ella Veenstra[2] gets out of bed, and walks to her bathroom. Ella, as her care workers affectively call her, is living with Alzheimer's disease in a Dutch sub-urban care home called 'Zonneweide'.[3] She moved here six years ago, when she was no longer able to manage by herself. That Ms Veenstra gets up in the morning is the result of a lot of work on the part of her care workers. Every day anew, when asked to get up, she insists on staying in bed, stating that she has a headache. Indeed, Ms Veenstra is known to have had migraines for most of her life and is given a light pain killer every morning and 'more if necessary'. However, so her care workers tell me, her headaches 'may have become a bit of an excuse to not get up'. Her caregivers check her perspiration and her eyes to determine when she 'really' has a headache. When the care worker on duty thinks she does not, she[4] starts to encourage Ms Veenstra to get up, acting on the team's agreement that it is best for Ms Veenstra to get out of bed: once she is up, she eats with the other residents and forgets about wanting to stay in bed.

A. Driessen (✉)
Amsterdam Institute for Social Science Research (AISSR), University of Amsterdam, Amsterdam, The Netherlands

© The Author(s) 2018
F. Krause, J. Boldt (eds.), *Care in Healthcare*,
https://doi.org/10.1007/978-3-319-61291-1_7

> Sometimes Ms Veenstra goes back to bed after breakfast, and her care givers agree that doing so should be allowed. In talking about situations like getting Ella up, care worker Anja tells me: 'This is the difficulty with care work, especially with people with dementia.' She gives me other examples: '[Another resident] always says "Let me stay in bed, let me stay in bed". [...] But she eats better when she is up—then she sits upright; she drinks better; she reads a paper and participates in activities. Then one sees that getting up has an added value. With people with dementia you typically have to make choices for them, because they cannot do that anymore.' I push the conversation: 'But they *do* make a choice, only not the one that is right in your eyes.' Anja retorts: 'I could follow [her] choice, but then I know I am not providing good care. [...].' I ask: 'So it is about good care?' upon which Anja answers: 'Yes, good care is the basis. Taking one shower per week is really the minimum. There is another lady who has a trauma from showering because she once stood under boiling hot water. In that case, she really does not have to shower; I'll wash her instead. [...] I would not coerce her to get into the shower.'

These stories are examples of situations that many caregivers working in dementia care homes will recognise immediately: the resident wants something that the care worker thinks is not good for her. In other words, what a resident wants (here, to stay in bed) does not always align with what the caregiver wants (here, if the resident does not seem to have a migraine, to get the resident up, and, ideally, for the resident to want this as well).[5]

While the tension between opposing desires is certainly not unique to dementia care, it is characteristic for care encounters with those living with decreasing mental capacities. With the progression of the dementia, the person living with the condition requires increasing levels of assistance to complete everyday bodily tasks: she will need more help with getting up and being washed and dressed. Some people simultaneously lose their awareness of the need to get up and keep clean. Although staying in bed and refraining from washing is possible for some days, doing so for longer may come to harm one's health and well-being. Therefore, accomplishing the tasks of getting residents up and washed falls to care workers. This sometimes results in situations in which residents refuse to get up, do not want a shower or want to wear their favourite shirt while their care worker finds it too dirty to wear.[6] Studies on care work have pointed out that care workers often call residents who do not want the same as themselves in activities of daily living (ADL) care encounters 'difficult' or exhibiting 'challenging behaviour' (e.g. Higgs and Gilleard 2015, pp. 89–90). But they frequently stop short at unpacking how this encounter plays out when it presents itself.

To want something is an expression of subjectivity, and being respected in one's desires is as much part of living a good life in a dementia care home as it is elsewhere. But how can we think about what residents want in cases which lead their care workers to assert that what a resident wants is not good for her? Indeed, if care were just about 'getting the job done' then the *way* it is done would not be relevant. In practice, however, this clearly matters. As care worker Cici remarked: 'As a normal human being you do not want to be forced all the time!' Similarly, one may not want to be left to one's fate all alone either. Indeed, there is a lot in between.

This is not to say that coercion or neglect never happens in care work. When Ms Lichthart woke up covered in her own faeces, but was nevertheless resisting a shower, two care workers held her in a tight grip while another washed her quickly. It seemed 'the only way to do this'. Ms Lichthart indeed needed a shower, but by washing her this way, what she wanted was overruled. Yet, rather than concluding that 'things are not going well in care' because these situations do occur, I want to emphasise here that such generalisations about care work miss something: they miss the work that care workers do on a daily basis to prevent these extreme measures. This work becomes most visible in situations in which what a resident wants is opposed to what a care worker wants.

Debates on the will are an obvious starting point to take a closer look at these situations. Thinking about the will has long been the domain of philosophers. In the most general sense, philosophers have understood the will as the '"faculty, or set of abilities, that yields the mental events involved in volition", where volition is understood to be "a mental event in the initiation of action"' (Brand 1995, p. 843 in Murphy and Throop 2010, p. 7). Debates on the topic have focused on the (in)compatibility of relative freedom and determinacy of human choice and action. Within these debates, moral philosophers attach particular value to the free will. After all, whether, or to what extent, we can act freely informs whether we have a choice to act in a good or bad way in the first place. Put differently, without a will that is free (at least to some degree), moral decision making is not possible.

Dementia care presents an interesting case to think about 'the will', as dementia is usually said to invalidate it altogether. For instance, Dutch law uses the term 'wilsonbekwaam' (which translates freely to 'will-incompetent'[7]) for those who are unable to understand or deliberate on information that is provided to them, who cannot make a decision and/or who no longer understand the consequences of their decisions (Rijksoverheid 2014). This legal category dismisses the person's will, making possible, for example, a person's admission to a nursing home against her will.[8]

The philosophical and legal accounts both reflect an understanding of the will as related to cognition and rationality. This understanding may be useful with regard to long-term decision making (which indeed becomes increasingly difficult for people with dementia with the progression of the condition). However, it is less helpful with regard to the 'daily wanting' on the dementia ward. Indeed, a lot is wanted on the dementia ward! How may we think about those situations?

Much anthropological writing can be read as a critique of the rational understanding of 'the will'. In using concepts such as agency, intentionality, motive, desire, wish and motivation, anthropologists are perhaps only implicitly speaking about the will, but nevertheless bring to light a complex interweaving with emotional and physical states. This literature provides a helpful background against which to rethink the will in relation to dementia and dementia care, and situations in which residents want something different than their caregivers want for them in particular. However, this body of work lacks a definitional consensus and thus a common ground for discussion. In their edited volume 'Toward an Anthropology of the Will', Keith Murphy and Jason Throop (2010) make considerable steps towards such a consensus. In his contribution to the volume, Jason Throop argues that the will is experienced as somehow one's own, goal-directed and effortful (2010, p. 34). While this is important when thinking about why what somebody wants cannot be simply overruled, Throop is right in suggesting that there is still

> a necessity of shifting from this descriptive phenomenological approach to willing to exploring how these various experiential correlates of willing may be differently organized, affected and expressed in the context of unfolding

social interaction, personal narratives, and reflections upon past, present and future experiences. (Throop 2010, p. 49)

In this chapter, I take up Throop's invitation to think further about 'willing' in interaction. However, as I discuss in more detail in the following paragraph, I focus on 'daily wanting' instead of willing, as it is worked upon in the context of unfolding sociomaterial interaction. Moreover, I ask what we may learn about good care from taking a closer look at these practices. Based on my ethnography[9] of ADL-care situations in which residents with dementia often want something other than what their caregivers think is good for them, I argue that, rather than coercing residents into doing whatever task is at hand, care workers attempt to align what residents' want with what they themselves want (for them). I propose the concept of 'sociomaterial will-work' to describe this work and reflect on its limits and implications. At the same time caregivers may come to want something else too; will-work can thus align the wanting of residents but also of their caregivers.

Work on Wanting: Sociomaterial Will-Work

Before going into the ethnography of ADL encounters in which wanting is aligned, I want to highlight two methodological interventions that I make with this chapter. Firstly, I contend that the term 'will' suggests a coherence that hides the relational nature of coming to want something. I therefore suggest that, rather than understanding the will as something we 'have', we should understand it as something we 'do' in unfolding sociomaterial interaction. Secondly, since my interest here is in understanding the alignment that is strived for in the process of wanting in dementia care settings *on a daily basis*, I differentiate between 'willing' and 'wanting'. I separate a more cognitive intending, pertaining to the realm of the legal and long-term decision making ('willing'), from a more immediate, emotionally and physically informed activity ('wanting'). I understand wanting[10] to be a fundamental expression of subjectivity, including activities such as desiring, longing, wishing and, significantly, not wanting, which is done in unfolding sociomaterial interaction on an everyday basis.

In defining the will as something we do in sociomaterial interaction, I align myself with the tradition of material semiotics, in which practices take central stage (Law 2009). I put my writings in conversation with the work on care practices (e.g. Jerak-Zuiderent 2015; Mol 2002; 2008; Mol et al. 2010; Moser 2010a, b; Van Hout et al. 2015; Vogel 2017). Within this tradition, I have been particularly inspired by the work of Jeannette Pols with patients in psychiatric and residential care. She draws our attention to the fact that residents of psychiatric nursing homes, rather than *saying* what they like, make their appreciations known by *enacting* them (Pols 2005). Positing that appreciations can be enacted means that they can be expressed both verbally as well as non-verbally. Any interaction may thus include gestures, facial expressions and actions. This is important when thinking about dementia, as most nursing home residents—whether aphasic, passive, confused or hallucinating—can and do express whether they want something or not. They may do so by softly uttering a 'yes', seeking company or trying to escape it, pushing their plate away or, indeed, by not heeding the call to get out of bed. This has a crucial methodological consequence: as residents *do* appreciations in situations that are co-produced by the material environment and other people, they may be observed.[11]

If wanting is *done*, as I suggest, in unfolding sociomaterial interaction, how it is then acted upon is almost inevitably an ethical and political question. As I have mentioned before, wanting is an essential expression of subjectivity, and is thus best respected and stimulated. Indeed, avoiding coercion was central to many conversations I had with care workers. They commonly held the understanding that in order to get residents to 'cooperate' [meewerken], 'urging [aandringen] is allowed, but coercing [dwingen] is not'.[12] Care workers also told me time and again that '[i]f a resident *really* does not want to do something, then she does not have to do it'. The distinction that is made between 'what a resident wants' and 'what a resident *really* wants' is an interesting one. Indeed, the word *really* indicates that what is wanted is—at least to some degree—flexible. It is this flexibility that is used to 'urge' residents. The exchange with Anja makes this visible: while she says she makes decisions for residents, she adapts her way of providing care to them, and what they 'really' want, or do not want. She thus strives to complete ADL-care without coercion or neglect: the resident who is traumatised from standing under boiling water does not *have* to shower, and Anja washes her by the sink instead. Indeed, care workers tried to negotiate with residents if they did not want to do a task the care givers asserted needed to be done. Care workers also often proved flexible in showering residents at another point in time and giving in to residents who, for instance, insisted on wearing certain clothes.

I propose to call the practices in which residents and care workers seek to (creatively) align what they both want 'sociomaterial will-work'.[13,14] I am indebted to three bodies of work for the concept. First, my choice of the word 'sociomaterial' builds on the material semiotic tradition. Herein, social and material 'aspects', previously separated in social sciences, 'get mixed up in ethnographic descriptions of the practices in which they are being handled' (Harbers et al. 2002, p. 208). Second, my choice for the word 'work' relies on theories of (interpersonal) body work (Gimlin 2007; Twigg et al. 2011; Twigg 2000; Wolkowitz 2002), emotional labour (Hochschild 1979, 1983) and sentimental work (Strauss et al. 1982). This literature emphasises the dual nature of these types of work (largely organised as 'women's work') as both a loving attitude and a form of (paid) labour. This insight informs the concept of will-work in significant ways: will-work is *work*; it takes time, effort, and skills, and it is a central aspect of care giving, which requires an attentive caregiver. The types of work described above and will-work can be highly entangled. Acknowledging this adds to a more complex understanding of what giving care to people with dementia entails. Third, the concept of will-work rests on the shoulders of feminist care ethicists (e.g. Gilligan 1982; Tronto 1993), who have advocated for an acknowledgement of peoples' dependence and interdependency on one another. Will-work is a deeply relational practice: in doing will-work care workers rely on relational knowledge, acquired in their everyday work with the same people, often for the duration of years. In the unfolding interactions, resident and care worker relate to one another. Care ethics has been critiqued by disability studies for rendering care receivers passive recipients of care (Williams 2001, pp. 478–479).[15] While existing power differences in the care encounter should not be disregarded, the concept of will-work is explicitly not applicable to the work of care workers only: care receiver's wanting may be aligned to having a shower, but the caregivers' wanting may also be aligned to flexibly adjust to what the care receiver wants. This could take the form of providing assistance with a shower later, asking another caregiver to step in or perhaps reconsidering whether the task at hand is necessary at all.

I contend that doing will-work (rather than neglecting or overruling residents' wanting) makes the caregivers' work good care. Good care includes being attentive to people's desires and striving 'to lighten what is heavy, and even if it fails it keeps on trying' (Mol et al. 2010, p. 14). Good dementia care, then, 'persistently strives to create conditions for and enable better interaction, and also to afford people living with dementia positions in which they can act and exert valued forms of subjectivity' (Moser 2010a, p. 295). Coercion or neglect forecloses opportunities for 'better interaction'. Through coercion, positions in which subjectivity can be exerted are not afforded, and wanting can, by definition, not be shared. If wanting cannot be done together, and cannot be aligned, it remains unilateral—which can be harmful in situation where one must agree and where there are power differences. In these situations, will-work aims to achieve what is good for those living with dementia (an assertion that often relies on professional knowledge) in a way that is pleasant for the resident as well as for the caregiver. At the same time, it must includes a reflecting upon whether the task at hand must be completed now, and in this particular way.

In the remaining pages, I describe the work care workers do on residents' wanting as (1) sculpting moods and emotions, (2) managing attention and (3) creative negotiation involving time and materialities.

Sculpting Moods and Emotions

The first way in which will-work is done, begins *before* something is wanted. Consider the following interview excerpt:

Annelieke:	Can you tell me something about ADL-care and dementia, and what is specific for people with dementia, particularly when compared to people with somatic complaints?
Leandra:	Specific? I think it differs, and depends on the person [you are dealing with] and how you deal with it. [...] I always adjust to how advanced someone is [in his/her dementia].
Annelieke:	Hmm. What do you mean? Or—what do you do?
Leandra:	You walk in [to the resident's room] and then you try to come in as 'cheerfully' [luchtig] as possible.

Annelieke: Do you mean like [happy tone of voice] 'Hallo'?

Leandra Yes, you try to brighten up the room when you walk in [het zonnetje in huiszijn]. I notice that Ms Koch, [...] when I go there and I am cheerful, then she also becomes cheerful. [I]magine you come in looking all serious, not even sad, but just neutral, [...] then she is already more sad. So, the emotion that you radiate, she magnifies that. [Sometimes] you notice that nothing works and that [the fact that she does not want to be washed] is due to her mood at that moment. [...] But I see that it works when I enter happily, because it relaxes her and she will allow me to do more.

This example shows Leandra doing will-work. She wants to shower Ms Koch.[16] In order to do this, she needs Ms Koch to *want* to shower, or at least to not refuse it. Leandra's initial use of the generic 'you' indicates that entering the room cheerfully is a more general way of approaching residents. But she then adjusts to the person herself and to the severity of the resident's condition, as is evidenced in Ms Koch's example. In other words, generalisations are not useful here. To get Ms Koch to want to shower, Leandra attempts to sculpt her mood. Although sometimes 'nothing works' and wanting remains not amenable to Leandra to work upon it, sometimes it *does* work: in those situations, Leandra's smile causes Ms Koch to 'also become cheerful', to 'magnify the emotion' and to relax. This, in turn, results in her allowing Leandra 'to do more', including giving her a shower.

In another example of this way of doing will-work, Joani often brought three cups of hot chocolate to Ms Veenstra along with her medicine. We drank the chocolate by her bedside together. Meanwhile, we talked about the weather or what we had done yesterday, or about the joint breakfast awaiting her downstairs. By doing this, Joani hoped to get Ms Veenstra into the mood for getting out of bed, and it often worked. In those cases, what Ms Veenstra wanted was aligned with Joani's desire for her to have breakfast, and for her to be with others.

Sculpting moods and emotions is one way to align wanting. Two important conclusions can be drawn from this. Firstly, the story affirms that moods and emotions cannot be separated from wanting.[17] Secondly, it shows will-work as a relational practice: Ms Koch and Leandra are responsive to one another's moods, smiles and tone of voice. Joani and Ms Veenstra first had a chat, after which wanting to get up could become a shared desire. Thirdly, materialities, such as cups of hot chocolate or breakfast, may be part of the attempt to align wanting.

Managing Attention

So far, I have described how care workers sculpt moods and emotions that then allow residents to want what care workers want for them. Sometimes, when Leandra enters the room cheerfully, Ms Koch 'magnifies the emotion'. Leandra's cheerfulness changes Ms Koch's mood and thus her willingness to take a shower. But 'coming in cheerfully' is not enough. What do care workers do to keep the wanting aligned once they walk through the door? Leandra engages in a second way of will-work after she has entered the room cheerfully:

Annelieke: Okay, […] you try to brighten up the room when you walk in. […] And then?

Leandra: And then you start instructing [the resident]: 'what are we going to do today' […] and instead of pausing for a long time afterwards [you] talk about other things and […] you keep control over the topic of conversation. You have the lead in what happens. […] Take Ms Stein, if you tell her 'Good morning, I will give you a nice wash', she will say 'yes, but but but […]'. But if you right away talk about something else, then the 'but but' that you could expect is over. Then she is already somewhere else. […] I say: 'How did you sleep?', 'Not so well'. Then I say 'How is that possible? Was it too warm? Was it too cold?' 'Well no, no, I don't know. I don't know'. 'Are you hungry?' 'Yes, I am quite hungry' 'Well, then I will [say] 'look, a wash cloth' or something, you know, 'Then you can have a nice breakfast. What would you like? White bread, brown bread? A whole conversation about what is about to happen. […] Well, then you are nicely engaged. I am too; I don't like saying nothing. So it is also nicer for […] me.

Leandra seems to imply that Ms Stein's cannot want something other than the tasks at hand—being washed while having a conversation. In other words, doing wanting (here, not wanting to shower) requires Ms Stein's attention. Doing will-work in this situation entails managing that attention: Leandra orients Ms Stein towards what they are going to do, away from not wanting to shower, and times her questions to 'keep control over the topic of conversation'. In doing so, Leandra keeps Ms Stein's 'yes but' at bay. By 'talking about something else', Leandra can distract Ms Stein from the task at hand and let it go almost unnoticed. Leandra thus prevents that Ms Stein comes to want something other than a shower. When Leandra 'has the lead in what happens', Ms Stein is 'already somewhere else' instead of in her rejection of the washing. Both are 'nicely engaged'. This affects Ms Stein positively: if she is off to a good start, she is more likely to enjoy the rest of her day as well.

In a similar vein, Anja manages the residents' attention by offering a choice about the timing of showering, rather than about showering itself:

Anja: My biggest trick is to give people *one* choice, no discussion. I ask [...]: 'would you like to shower now or in half an hour?' Then they feel like they have a say in it, although they do not [have a say about whether to actually have a shower or not] ... 'It would be nice if you would wear a clean shirt today. Do you want this one or that one?' (She holds up her hands as if she is holding two shirts next to each other.) Idem ditto with 'do you want to have a shower now or in thirty minutes?' In fact, they do not get a say. ... 'Yes...'; 'That one' (and she points to one of her hands with the imaginary shirt). It simply is a bath-day! Then [when I pose this question], they are often so overwhelmed, that they just come along. (Emphasis original)

Anja emphasises that, if she does not provide ADL-care, she says that she knows she is 'not providing good care'. Good care, as described by Anja here, means to make the resident want what Anja thinks is good for her. In providing a binary choice about timing, she offers the resident a *sense* of choice, yet makes sure that she chooses the shower, which Anja says is good for her.

Leandra and Anja manage the resident's attention to prevent that she may come to want something other than what they, as her care workers, contend is good for her. One could argue that these ways of doing will-work are manipulative.[18] If we consider the will to be a fixed entity, it may well be. But if, as I suggested, we see wanting as done in unfolding socio-material interaction (which may include cups of hot chocolate, smiles and a cheerful tone of voice, as well as attempts to keep control over the conversation), we can understand the attempts to manage attention as attempts to turn wanting into a *relational* activity, rather than an individual one: Care workers take what residents want as something that can be worked upon and made relational in the care encounter. In doing so, care workers take residents' wanting seriously in that it cannot simply be overruled, but neither can it be taken to be a fixed entity which cannot be changed. Rather than forcing their will upon residents, care workers remain in conversation. They offer a sense of choice where perhaps there is none (as Anja put it, it may be 'simply a bath-day'![19]), but do not merely impose something on the resident. Managing attention is thus part of the larger attempt to align wanting in a way that ensures that care tasks that care workers deem necessary get done, in a way that is as pleasant as possible for both people involved. At best, both are 'nicely engaged'.

Creative Negotiation Involving Time and Materialities

Leandra enters the room in a friendly mood. She controls the conversation and diverts the residents' attention away from coming to want something other than the care task at hand. Anja offers a choice on time, rather than on the task itself. These are ways to work on residents' wanting *before* they fixate on wanting something. In this section I describe how care workers attempt to modify what a resident wants when a resident already expressed a wanting before it could be sculpted. I call this work 'creative negotiation'.[20]

First and foremost, care workers ask residents for their 'cooperation' in the care activity. If this does not work, care workers also reason with residents, either jokingly or seriously. Herein they often argue based on visible materialities in the present ('Look, your shirt is dirty'), relating them to what is to be done now ('Let's put on a clean shirt') or in the near future ('Don't you want to look clean when your family visits this afternoon?'). These strategies seem to appeal to a cognitive willing (resonating the philosophical understanding of the will)—which is precisely what residents in the early stages of dementia seem to be losing grip on—but not to an emotional wanting. Indeed, these strategies do not work with all residents, and certainly not every time.

If reasoning does not work, there are other strategies. Care workers, for instance, play with the timing of caregiving. When Mr Bakker does not want to get up, Joani often asks: 'Would you like me to come back in half an hour?' If he agrees, she simply helps the residents in a different order, creating a temporary alignment between what she and Mr Bakker want: to not shower (just yet). Mr Bakker is often willing to get up after half an hour or so, perhaps having fulfilled his desire to stay in bed longer, or perhaps having forgotten his reluctance to get up in the first place. As such, time helps in aligning wanting.[21]

When continuing attempts to align the residents' wanting with their own become too challenging, care workers sometimes call upon a colleague to take over. Care workers remain patient with the resident by putting space between themselves and a resident whose wanting remained not amenable to negotiation. Sometimes a specific colleague is asked. This once again highlights the relational nature of will-work: if a care worker gets along well with a resident, aligning wanting becomes easier to do. For instance, when nobody can get Ms Veenstra out of bed and Lucia is working that day, her colleagues ask her to come and help. Lucia can 'pull off' a stricter approach and 'get away with it'. She can tell Ms Veenstra: 'My dear, you stink, you must get up'. Anja said: 'Ms Veenstra would get angry at any other care worker for saying anything of the sort, but she *loves* Lucia'.

Like the cups of hot chocolate worked for sculpting wanting, materialities can also play a role in creative negotiation. Take the case of Mr Bakker. Convincing Mr Bakker to wear clean clothes and to take a shower poses a challenge every day. He is known to feel cold and claustrophobic, so that the bathroom door cannot be closed to make him feel warmer.

Mr Bakker has vascular dementia and is aphasic: he can utter short sentences, with the occasional loss of a word. Not being able to find and understand words frustrates Mr Bakker and reasoning is likely to upset him. Joani is particularly skilled[22] in finding alternatives to reasoning by 'creatively negotiating' with him, not only verbally, but also non-verbally: one day, when faced with his refusal to take a shower, she gave him a foot bath. Then he wanted the shower.

In talking about this situation, Joani and I offered differing explanations for why the foot bath had worked. I suspected that giving Mr Bakker the foot bath made him feel less cold, undoing his reason to refuse the shower. Joani said: 'The foot bath gets him out of his head. If he puts his feet in warm water—maybe he remembers something, that he walks down the beach for instance—but once his feet feel the warm water, he would have to hold onto his thoughts of "not wanting to shower" *very* rigidly'. Joani imagines that the sensation of warm water on his feet reminds Mr Bakker of the ocean. This goes further than to *think* about the ocean: the water makes him *feel* something he has felt before and thus conjures up (hopefully happy) memories. This pleasant feeling, then, in her understanding, made him let go of his opposition to showering.

How the foot bath 'really' changed Mr Bakker's wanting is up for speculation. But two other points illustrate my argument about daily wanting and will-work here. Firstly, wanting something seems highly entangled with the feeling body, which may then be 'tinkered with' (cf. Mol et al. 2010) in the context of the care relationship. In doing will-work, the feeling body may be skilfully appealed to. Secondly, not only interactions between people sculpt or prevent a specific wanting, but so do non-human actors: here, work on Mr Bakker's wanting required a foot bath. If the foot bath had not been part of the encounter, Joani could have tried cheering up Mr Bakker, arranging another time slot for his care or asking one of her colleagues to take over. But instead, the will-work was 'delegated' (Latour 1988, p. 299) to the foot bath. Herewith, it becomes clear that will-work can be done involving objects: the foot bath creates the material conditions that work upon what Mr Bakker enjoys, and in doing so, change what Mr Bakker wanted. The foot bath opened up an avenue for Mr Bakker to want a shower.

Conclusion

In this chapter, I set out to explore in more detail the way in which daily wanting is worked upon in the context of unfolding sociomaterial interaction in residential dementia care, and I asked what we may learn about good care from taking a closer look at these practices. I stated that wanting is an expression of subjectivity, and being respected in this is a prerequisite for living a good life with dementia. At the same time, wanting something is a relational process. How it is acted upon thus is an ethical and political question. Nobody wants to constantly be overruled by another person, and indeed much work goes into avoiding coercing somebody. To describe what is done instead, I coined the term 'sociomaterial will-work'. The concept highlights care workers' and residents' attempts to align the other's wanting with their own as a form of labour and as dependent on sociomaterial relations. I described care workers doing will-work by (1) sculpting moods and emotions, (2) managing attention and (3) creative negotiation involving time and materialities. With smiles, cups of hot chocolate and foot baths, changes to the order in which care is provided and to who shows up at a resident's bed, care workers strive for a positive way of relating—of being 'nicely engaged' in conversation and activity. Will-work ventures into the space between doing nothing and exerting force. It is the 'urging' that care workers name when seeking alternatives for coercion and neglect. I have argued that this aligning residents' wanting makes the caregivers' work good care.

I have offered an alternative understanding of the will—namely as something that is 'done' in sociomaterial interaction, in which it can be aligned by making it relational. Indeed, instead of dismissing 'daily wanting' of those living with dementia, my analysis enables thinking about it. At the same time, the finding that moods and the feeling body can be appealed to in care encounters and that materialities can be used in creative negotiation with residents, offers new ways of thinking about what good care may entail in situations in which residents want something that their care workers understand as 'not good' for them. As such, my contribution is one that can inform care practice.

Some may say I have painted a rather ideal picture. What can be done when 'nothing works', which, as Leandra noted, sometimes happens? In these cases, will-work seems to hit its limit and coercion may seem the only way to get a task done (we may think again of Ms Lichthart, who, covered in faeces, resisted a shower). It is important not to forget that people living with dementia, who are often aphasic and have a fragmented memory, are particularly vulnerable to maltreatment and situations in which what they want (or resist) is overruled. Doing will-work requires the continuous reflection upon the fine line between 'urging' and 'coercing'. Once, when Ms Veenstra did not want to get out of bed, her care worker Linda turned on the TV, radio and shower, and pulled away her blankets. These were trying moments of participant observation, as being there without doing anything about it made me complicit. Upon my inquiry why Linda did this, she explained: 'This will annoy her so much that she will get up. She is better off if she gets up and eats something'. Paradoxically, Linda was convinced that what she was doing was caring. The example shows that a care worker can easily abuse his or her power, even if the actions are based on the idea that the resident in question is 'better off' like this. But the way in which care tasks are achieved matters. Coercion, neglect and incisive refusal leave no room for alignment in wanting. Wanting, in those situations, remains unilateral and cannot be shared. Although coercion does indeed result in Ms Veenstra getting up, *how* this is achieved imposes what Linda wants on her; wanting, instead of being done together, remains unilateral. Indeed, it is dubious whether this can still be called good care.

I contend that will-work has failed when a resident is coerced into doing something. Sociomaterial will-work makes good care only if care workers continue to attempt to align residents' wanting with what they think is good for them, after critically reflecting on the question whether this is indeed so. If will-work fails, coercion and neglect remain tragic occurrences. But if given enough time, trust and support, care workers doing will-work may indeed realise the proverbial 'otherwise' (Star 1990, pp. 89–90), enabling residents like Ms Lichthart to *want* the shower that they need.

I do not want to make it seem that care work is easy. On the contrary, I explicitly want to acknowledge that persistent tinkering without 'successes' requires a lot of patience, which under trying circumstances is sometimes sheer impossible. This is why time, energy and motivation are indeed essential for retaining the flexibility that is needed to do will-work in delicate care situations with frail and fragile residents. Cuts to staff, the subsequent increase in work load and a lack of trust within care teams are detrimental to the care staff's ability to do good care. Under such circumstances, residents such as Ms Lichthart covered in faeces are sometimes forced to shower. At the same time, however, good care is already being done. I have taken all examples presented in this chapter from what I have seen in the care homes where I conducted my research. In writing about these, rather than about the situations in which care falls short, I hope to give this work the attention it deserves. I use these examples to hold up to others: that way, what already works well, can be done more often.

Notes

1. Like any text, this text is the result of a collaborative effort. I would like to extend my gratitude to the Gieskes-Strijbis Fonds for funding this research. I owe my deepest thanks to the care institutions which granted me access for my fieldwork, and the care professionals and residents who gave so much of their time to me, and patiently took me along in their daily life and work. In particular, I would like to thank the organisers of the summer school that led to this book, Joachim Boldt and Franziska Krause, and to the summer school's participants, whom I can now proudly call my esteemed co-authors and friends. Special thanks go to Patrick McKearney and my dear colleagues at the University of Amsterdam, of whom I want to mention in particular Willemijn Krebbekx, Else Vogel, Lex Kuiper, Annekatrin Skeide, my in the Anthropology of Care research group Silke Hoppe, Laura Vermeulen, Natashe Lemos Dekker and Susanne van den Buusethe members of the Writing Care Seminar and the Walking Seminar Amsterdam. Daniel Guinness, thank you for editing my English! Lastly, but with emphasis, I want to thank my supervisors at the University of Amsterdam: Anne-Mei The for giving me the opportunity to do this research, and Jeannette Pols and Kristine Krause for being such a big source of inspiration and support throughout the research and writing process.
2. All names used in this chapter, for sites as well as interlocutors, are pseudonyms.

3. 'Zonneweide' (a fictitious name) is one of three care homes in which I conducted ethnographic fieldwork. It is a care home in a sub-urban area in the Netherlands and home to 50 people with a wide variety of diagnoses. Fifteen of them live on the floor reserved for people with early stage dementia, although, if possible, residents live here until they pass away. Recent changes in Dutch health care policy resulted in the closing of many of the care homes that are providing care to people with 'lower' care needs. Those that remain open, like Zonneweide, are increasingly providing care to people with 'higher' care needs, including those in the later stages of dementia.
4. For purposes of legibility, I use the female pronoun to refer to residents and care workers in general.
5. The caregivers' reasons to want something pertain to achieving a high level of well-being for the resident in question, and thus doing their job well. In a way, it is thus what professional caregivers want for residents *and* for themselves. If wanting can be aligned, the situation is significantly more pleasant for both parties involved.
6. In this chapter, I focused on those situations in which residents want something else than the care worker(s) in care encounters that centre around activities of daily living (ADL). These particular situations are characterised mostly by a resident *not* wanting to do what the care worker has to 'get done': getting residents up, bathing and dressing them. I have chosen these situations because they most clearly bring out how wanting is negotiated in care encounters. However, in focusing on ADL care, my writing seems to suggest that residents merely refuse and hardly actively want anything. This is not the case in practice: residents want many things, some of which are equally 'problematic' for care workers (such as wanting to go home, contiuously wanting to go to the toilet or desiring intimacy with other residents. In those situations the family's wishes may also play an important role, a party that I have not been able to include in this chapter). By the same token, the situations in which residents do not necessarily want anything, but care workers stimulate them to do so, are left out. Both this 'wanting something' and the 'activation to want something' warrant further exploration.
7. In English, a person is said to no longer have legal capacity or to be (legally) incapacitated.
8. The issue of admitting somebody to a nursing home against her will is more complex than can be accounted for within the scope of this chapter. It must be noted here, however, that admission against somebody's

will is only possible if (a) somebody is endangering her own or other peoples' safety, (b) this situation cannot be resolved without admission to a nursing home and (c) a BOPZ-indication is assigned [a designation assigned to the person by a medical professional under the law of 'Bijzondere Opnemingen in Psychiatrische Ziekenhuizen' (Special admissions in psychiatric hospitals)] (cf. Rijksoverheid n.d.).

9. I build my argument with ethnographic material that I gathered during 14 months of fieldwork in three Dutch care institutions between summer 2013 and fall 2015. In all three care institutions I met the residents, and observed and participated in their daily activities. Additionally, I observed and participated in care practices, helping care workers with their ADL-tasks on the wards during day, evening and night shifts. I conducted interviews with carers and family members. The analysis consisted of a careful readings and re-readings of all interview transcripts and field notes. I coded the data for recurring themes, using NVivo qualitative data analysis software. One of these themes is 'daily wanting' on the ward and how it was negotiated in care encounters, the analysis of which I present in this chapter. Ethical consent for the research was obtained from the Anthropology Ethics Board of the University of Amsterdam.
10. I deliberately choose the term 'wanting' over 'agency'. While agency, most generally, refers to the 'socioculturally mediated capacity to act' (Ahearn 2001, p. 112), hence *potentialities* of action, I here discuss actual practices in which wanting is *done*, and thus actually takes place.
11. This approach is useful to make visible how people with dementia who can no longer express themselves in verbally coherent ways, are nevertheless actors in the world. However, it simultaneously makes invisible mixed motives and intentions. If, for example, a resident steps into the shower upon the urging of her care worker, this action could, instead of an enactment of the will, also be a way to please her, or to put an end to the conversation. These considerations cannot be grasped through the approach chosen.
12. The statement can be said to reflect a wider shift away from coercive measures in Dutch health care, and may thus have been related to the language used in culture change programmes aiming to change care workers' attitude towards the use of coercion. At the same time, neglect, or the milder form of ignoring somebody, was less discussed. These situations (for instance, when a resident indicates that she wants to use the toilet, but care workers assert that 'she does not really need to go, she just *thinks* she does') merit more analysis.

13. For purposes of brevity, I hereafter use 'will-work'.
14. I chose to call the practice 'will-work' rather than 'wanting-work' because it allows me to put my writings in conversation with philosophical work on the will.
15. Interestingly, disability studies itself has been critiqued for putting care recipients into the same position (Winance 2010, p. 95).
16. For a wonderful analysis of repertoires in washing practices, see Jeannette Pols's 'Washing the citizen' (Pols 2006).
17. This illustrates the entanglement of will-work and emotional labour, defined by Arlie Hochschild as the 'management of feeling to create a publicly observable facial and bodily display' (Hochschild 1983, footnote p. 7) which 'requires one to induce or suppress feeling in order to sustain the outward countenance that produces the proper state of mind in others' (ibid., p. 7). Here, Leandra manages her own facial display to produce a happy state of mind in Ms Koch, who is then more likely to want a shower.
18. For an interesting reflection on deception and dementia, see 'Nothing but the truth? On truth and deception in dementia care' (Schermer 2007).
19. On a critical note: it is important that care workers keep asking themselves whether the resident *really* cannot skip the shower, or *really* does not want to shower—if the answer is no to both, then the shower may just be postponed, therein aligning the care worker's wanting with what the resident wants.
20. It goes without saying that the examples of creative negotiation provided here are not an exhaustive list. Whenever one 'way of doing things' did not work, care workers mostly tried another one, or combined them creatively. Therefore the list should not be seen as a scheme of possible actions, but rather to give an idea of how care workers improvise in situations in which residents' wanting does not align with what caregivers believes to be good for the resident (and thus with what the care worker would want the residents to want as well).
21. Interestingly, asking and rearranging the order in which residents are helped during the morning shift can become part of the daily routine too, without clashing with the efficiency-based logic of work in today's Dutch care homes. Indeed, investing time in doing will-work may thus even contribute to efficiency in some instances. As a care worker told me in response to a presentation of this chapter during a 'Dialogue meeting' [Dialoogbijeenkomst] organised by the Long Term Care and Dementia

research team I am part of, if a resident does not want to get dressed, time may be best spent 'seducing' that person into wanting to get dressed, rather than spending time in forcing the person into her clothes, as the latter action may be less pleasant for caregiver and care receiver, as well as more time consuming.

22. Clearly, it is necessary to take into account that these are largely personal and cannot be transferred from one care worker to another in every case. Indeed, not all care workers put as much creativity into the negotiation with residents. For instance, when Joani told Lucia about the foot bath she had given to Mr Bakker, Lucia replied 'I am not going to do *that!*'.

References

Ahearn, L. M. (2001). Language and Agency. *Annual Review of Anthropology, 30*, 109–137.

Brand, M. (1995). *Volition. The Cambridge Dictionary of Philosophy*. Cambridge: Cambridge University Press.

Gilligan, C. (1982). *In a Different Voice: Psychological Theory and Women's Development*. Cambridge: Harvard University Press.

Gimlin, D. (2007). What Is "Body Work"? A Review of the Literature. *Sociology Compass, 1*(1), 353–370.

Harbers, H., Mol, A., & Stollmeyer, A. (2002). Food Matters. *Theory, Culture & Society, 19*(5/6), 207–226.

Higgs, P., & Gilleard, C. (2015). *Rethinking Old Age: Theorising the Fourth Age*. London: Palgrave Macmillan.

Hochschild, A. R. (1979). Emotion Work, Feeling Rules, and Social Structure. *American Journal of Sociology, 85*(3), 551–575.

Hochschild, A. R. (1983). *The Managed Heart: Commercialization of Human Feeling*. Berkeley: University of California Press.

Jerak-Zuiderent, S. (2015). Accountability from Somewhere and for Someone: Relating with Care. *Science as Culture, 24*(4), 412–435.

Latour, B. (1988). Mixing Humans and Nonhumans Together: The Sociology of a Door-Closer. *Social Problems, 35*(3), 298–310.

Law, J. (2009). Actor Network Theory and Material Semiotics. In B. S. Turner (Ed.), *The New Blackwell Companion to Social Theory* (pp. 141–158). Oxford: Wiley-Blackwell.

Mol, A. (2002). *The Body Multiple. Ontology in Medical Practice*. Durham: Duke University Press.

Mol, A. (2008). *The Logic of Care: Health and the Problem of Patient Choice*. New York: Routledge.

Mol, A., Moser, I., & Pols, J. (Eds.). (2010). *Care in Practice: On Tinkering in Clinics, Homes and Farms*. Bielefeld: Transcript.

Moser, I. (2010a). Perhaps Tears Should Not Be Counted but Wiped Away: On Quality and Improvement in Dementia Care. In A. Mol, I. Moser, & J. Pols (Eds.), *Care in Practice: On Tinkering in Clinics, Homes and Farms* (pp. 277–322). Bielefeld: Transcript.

Moser, I. (2010b). Dementia and the Limits to Life: Anthropological Sensibilities, STS Interferences, and Possibilities for Action in Care. *Science, Technology, & Human Values, 36*(5), 704–722.

Murphy, K. M., & Throop, C. J. (Eds.). (2010). *Toward an Anthropology of the Will*. Stanford: Stanford University Press.

Pols, J. (2005). Enacting Appreciations: Beyond the Patient Perspective. *Health Care Analysis, 13*(3), 203–221.

Pols, J. (2006). Washing the Citizen: Washing, Cleanliness and Citizenship in Mental Health Care. *Culture, Medicine and Psychiatry, 30*(1), 77–104.

Rijksoverheid. (2014). Dwang in de zorg bij geheugenproblemen (dementie): wilsonbekwaam. *Dwangindezorg.nl*. Retrieved from https://www.dwangindezorg.nl/begrippenlijst/wilsonbekwaam

Rijksoverheid. (n.d.). Gedwongen opname in de zorg. *Rijksoverheid.nl*. Retrieved March 31, 2016, from https://www.rijksoverheid.nl/onderwerpen/geestelijke-gezondheidszorg/inhoud/gedwongen-opname-en-dwang-in-de-zorg

Schermer, M. (2007). Nothing but the Truth? On Truth and Deception in Dementia Care. *Bioethics, 21*(1), 13–22.

Star, S. L. (1990). Power, Technology and the Phenomenology of Conventions: On Being Allergic to Onions. *Sociological Review, 38(S1)*, 26–56.

Strauss, A., Fagerhaugh, S., Suczek, B., & Wiener, C. (1982). Sentimental Work in the Technologized Hospital. *Sociology of Health and Illness, 4*(3), 254–278.

Throop, C. J. (2010). In the Midst of Action. In K. M. Murphy & C. J. Throop (Eds.), *Toward an Anthropology of the Will* (pp. 24–49). Stanford: Stanford University Press.

Tronto, J. (1993). *Moral Boundaries: A Political Argument for an Ethic of Care*. London: Routledge.

Twigg, J. (2000). Carework as a Form of Bodywork. *Ageing and Society, 20*(4), 389–411.

Twigg, J., Wolkowitz, C., Cohen, R. L., & Nettleton, S. (2011). Conceptualising Body Work in Health and Social Care. *Sociology of Health & Illness, 33*(2), 171–188.

Van Hout, A., Pols, J., & Willems, D. (2015). Shining Trinkets and Unkempt Gardens: On the Materiality of Care. *Sociology of Health & Illness, 37*(8), 1206–1217.

Vogel, E. (2017). Hungers that Need Feeding: On the Normativity of Mindful Nourishment. *Anthropology & Medicine*, 1–15. doi:10.1080/13648470.2016.1276322.

Williams, F. (2001). In and Beyond New Labour: Towards a New Political Ethics of Care. *Critical Social Policy, 21*(4), 467–493.

Winance, M. (2010). Care and Disability: Practices of Experimenting, Tinkering with, and Arranging People and Technical Aids. In A. Mol, I. Moser, & J. Pols (Eds.), *Care in Practice: On Tinkering in Clinics, Homes and Farms* (pp. 93–117). Bielefeld: Transcript.

Wolkowitz, C. (2002). The Social Relations of Body Work. *Work, Employment and Society, 16*(3), 497–510.

Open Access This chapter is licensed under the terms of the Creative Commons Attribution 4.0 International License (http://creativecommons.org/licenses/by/4.0/), which permits use, sharing, adaptation, distribution and reproduction in any medium or format, as long as you give appropriate credit to the original author(s) and the source, provide a link to the Creative Commons license and indicate if changes were made.

The images or other third party material in this chapter are included in the chapter's Creative Commons license, unless indicated otherwise in a credit line to the material. If material is not included in the chapter's Creative Commons license and your intended use is not permitted by statutory regulation or exceeds the permitted use, you will need to obtain permission directly from the copyright holder.

The Dementia Village: Between Community and Society

Tobias Haeusermann

Introduction

The modern diagnosis of dementia has come to correspond with a number of connotations associated with old age: madness, incapacitation and psychological and social death.[1] Most people have heard of dementia, as basic disease facts and the factors that supposedly trigger or prevent it have been widely reported for decades, either reliably quoted or flagrantly misquoted. In biomedical terms, dementia is not a disease, but a syndrome produced in large part by diseases such as Alzheimer's, Parkinson's and vascular disease, to name merely a few (Haeusermann 2017). It is a cluster of symptoms and signs linked to the deterioration of cognitive abilities as a person ages. The word itself stems from the Latin *demens*, for "mad"—or, more accurately, "de-" + "mind" (*mens*)—and according to the *Diagnostic and Statistical Manual of Mental Disorders IV* (DSM-IV),

T. Haeusermann (✉)
Epidemiology, Biostatistics & Prevention Institute (EBPI), University of Zürich, Zürich, Switzerland

Department of Sociology, University of Cambridge, Cambridge, UK

© The Author(s) 2018
F. Krause, J. Boldt (eds.), *Care in Healthcare*,
https://doi.org/10.1007/978-3-319-61291-1_8

it may be caused or characterised by: "The development of multiple cognitive deficits manifested by both (1) memory impairment[2] [...] and (2) one or more of the following cognitive disturbances: (a) aphasia,[3] (b) apraxia,[4] (c) agnosia,[5] (d) disturbance in executive functioning"[6] (Weiner and Lipton 2009, p. 47). The term "dementia" thus encapsulates a collection of symptoms resulting from a progressive deterioration of cognitive function that cannot be accounted for by normal ageing and that have an impact on day-to-day activities (Ballard and Bannister 2010).

In their heyday, large-scale nursing homes provided a domestic space for the elderly in cognitive and physical decline. Yet they were dominated by officialdom and adherence to acute care protocols. As many critics have rightly pointed out,[7] such institutions did not always benefit their residents, especially those suffering from mental conditions. With time, the call for more individualistic and person-centred approaches was heard and new care models emerged. The initiation of a pioneering care facility, the Dutch Hogewey nursing home, strikingly embodies this shift. At its opening in 2009, it was the world's first and only village for residents with dementia. It was touted as a place where people could live and die in a communal setting, stripped of the impersonal hospital feel and clinical smell that most care homes still exude.[8]

The idea that it is more harmonious to live amongst primary groups in old age suggests itself intuitively. The significant media attention and conversations in geriatric circles surrounding the opening of the care villages made this plain.[9] Even before the popular media had shown interest, the concept caught attention in geriatric research circles.[10] Over the course of its first years and in response to the heightened media attention and the numerous requests from the geriatric community, the village offered one-day workshops for groups of one to five visitors. In its first years, the home became a Mecca for tour groups from all across the globe, and the home's administration decided to convert this rising public interest into monetary gain. Having heard of the new Dutch dementia village model, a team of employees of the Julius Tönebön Foundation in Hamelin, Germany, was sent to the Netherlands to learn more about the new approach with a view to incorporating their findings into a new project in Hamelin. Between May and December 2014, I conducted ethnographic research in the new German dementia village. This included a four-month period of intensive study, during which I lived in Hamelin. I spent nearly every day at the village, observing the typical daily activities and assisting the carers in their care routine. In August of that year, I accompanied the night shift workers for one month in order to gain insight into the village's night-time care activities. In total, I observed approximately 650 hours of care work, which entailed countless conversations with carers, residents and administrators, and attended around 60 handover meetings.[11]

The following paper draws on these experiences. It begins with an introduction to Germany's first dementia village *Tönbeön am See*, its setting and environment, the village's foundation, as well as the home's care philosophy. Throughout, I connect ethnographic observations with the broader events and developments. What follows is a discussion about the care village concept. I frame this discussion by examining the fundamental ambivalence that is inherent in the creation of a dementia village, situation its modern forms between the competing ideals illustrated by the concepts of *Gemeinschaft* (community) and *Gesellschaft* (society). Can these two concepts be combined? To offer some tentative answers, I explore how the notion of dementia manifests itself in real life and in the everyday behaviour of the village's residents, their families and the care takers.[12] I place dementia care at the centre of my analysis. I explore how dementia is experienced, controlled and managed within a distinct socio-cultural environment, at a distinct historical moment and within a specific body of knowledge available at the time. As such, this work's purpose lies in bringing light to the local dynamics and practices by which people with dementia, their families and their care takers are reciprocally and actively moulded into Germany's first dementia village. On a broader scale, this paper launches a more general discussion on ageing in contemporary society and shows how our representations of dementia and the ensuing care practices are largely determined by the social and cultural context.

The German Village

Tönebön am See is designed to provide a home for people in cognitive decline. Divided into four self-organised communities, it follows the principle of a manageable life world. The village lies in Hamelin, the capital of the district of Hamelin-Pyrmont, with a population of roughly 60,000. Around 200 kilometres east of the Dutch border and a half hour drive southwest of Hannover in northwest Germany, it is tucked away in hills and acts as a gateway to the neighbouring Weserbergland Mountains. The latter are a popular destination for both hikers and cyclists, though the town attracts most of its tourists thanks to its legendary Pied Piper folk tale. The legend tells a story, partially rooted in fact, that took place in the town during the thirteenth century. The Brothers Grimm brought it into worldwide prominence and it formed the subject of renowned poems by Goethe.[13] That Germany's first dementia village emerged from the birthplace of the Pied Piper tale is not devoid of irony.[14] While many tourists enjoy revelling in the thicket of Hamelin's history, it seems to be once again a lack of young persons that concerns the town and Germany as a whole. Yet a new and additional loss is emerging: the loss of mind and memory; and a variety of organisations and agents are offering their help and expertise.

The Julius Tönebön Foundation owns and manages the new dementia village. For over 60 years, the foundation has been active in the care business. They are, by their own valuation (and backed by official and semi-official comparison services), the regional market leader in the care home sector (Focus 2012). Based on their long-standing experience with dementia sufferers in their main care home, which is also situated in Hamelin and where the care recipients live in 3 residential groups of 18 residents each, it was decided that, ideally, the resident groups should be smaller. Moreover, it was thought that the common areas ought to offer more living space to cater for the residents' needs for intimacy, social proximity and security (Tönebön Stiftung 2016). Having heard of the new Dutch dementia village model, a team of employees was sent to the Netherlands to learn more about the new approach and how they could incorporate their findings into a new project in Hamelin. This resulted in four houses, all decorated in different colours and themes. Surrounded by a fenced-off space for 52 residents in total, the houses were intended to allow residents to feel at home away from their former homes. The home's administration defines the main care duties as caring and catering to the residents' physiological needs with food, drink and adequate housing. Meanwhile, their safety is protected by freedom from threats and economic deprivation, whereas their relational needs are met by the sense of belonging and affection offered through friendship, love and social interactions. Moreover, carers are instructed to approach residents with respect and to support their existing abilities. The residents, in turn, are expected to experience appreciation and feel self-esteem. In order to achieve this goal, the staff determine each resident's resources, nurture their remaining skills and look for ways in which each resident can compensate for deficient abilities by intervening individually and keeping in mind the specific situation. In line with these objectives, the residents' psychological and emotional needs take priority over physical care.[15]

Coming Home

I first found my way to the home on a hot and humid summer day. The home is difficult to reach by public transport. A bus stop is planned close by, but for now, a car is the primary and most sensible means of transport for visitors and staff. Some staff members who live in the vicinity, I later learned, cycle to work if the weather allows for it. I had thus decided to walk and was running late, as I had got lost in one of the many labyrinthine allotment gardens of Hamelin's outskirts. I frantically asked for directions, though no one I encountered could point me to the home. "A brain is a terrible thing to watch waste away", uttered a middle-aged woman, while clearing her neatly trimmed flower garden of weeds. "Good luck with your work, it is important to find a cure". Without a compass and a map, but thankfully able to speak the local language, I could only imagine the disorientation in time and place experienced by some residents every day. It could lead to a sense of panic, even eased by the certainty that it will pass. After a few detours through a web of footpaths, it did pass and I eventually stumbled upon the recently completed construction site. So new were its buildings that I could still smell the polished wood.

As I passed the entrance area and what turned out to be the home manager's office, I walked up to the reception desk, which was staffed by a receptionist. She was chatting amicably with a person who seemed to be a resident's family member. To my left I saw a café and a small supermarket.

The latter has been deemed an integral part of the dementia village concept, as it allows for a touch of normality. The supermarket is meant to distract from the clinical and cold ambiance commonly found in other care homes. Staffed by the receptionist, it is primarily open for residents who come accompanied with a carer. No money ever changes hands; the range of goods is limited to the residents' everyday dietary needs and some basic toiletries. Meanwhile, the café welcomes residents and guests alike. It offers a cosy retreat overseeing and giving access to the sensory garden, and, on occasion, is used for events and festivals. "Hello, Doctor Häusermann, we have been expecting you", the receptionist said. I greeted her and proceeded to inform her that I was not a doctor. The incident reminded me of the widely held German belief in authority and hierarchy. With half of my sentence still stuck deep within me, a resident scurried by and left the building. "Oh, would you mind running after Mrs Weber[16] and telling her to come back inside?" the receptionist asked calmly but sternly.

I ran after Mrs Weber and barely managed to catch up with her. Once I did, she finally came to a stop. She now stood in the parking area looking all around her, perplexed. Oblivious to my presence, she quietly mumbled some words to herself. I tentatively approached her, tapping her shoulder and introducing myself. She looked at me with tears in her eyes. With a soft and strained voice, she informed me that she was on her way home. I tried to convince her to walk back with me. While I spoke, she squinted her eyes, as though she were trying to decipher what I was saying. Then there was silence. Undoubtedly, I was having my first encounter with the slippery sense of truth in a world that, according to the media's imagination, produces a feigned reality. Steeped in yearning and in a dizzying and disorientated tone, Mrs Weber informed me that she was meant to meet her daughter for dinner and was already running late. She walked another couple of steps towards the cars, wistfully looking around as though she were selecting her vehicle of choice. I told her that dinner would be in the home tonight, which was true. But I lied when I was asked if I would call her daughter to let her know about the change of plans. "Do you know my daughter?", she asked gingerly. I said I did and would call her. She gave me a fleeting smile through her tears but did not seem fully convinced. I felt her determination. After repeating,

"Let's go back inside where it's not as hot", I gave her a squeeze on her arm, after which she reluctantly followed me back inside. As I stood with her in front of the reception desk, elbow-to-elbow, she looked at me with a lively face. "Thank you!" she said and, in a perfectly coherent sentence, added, "It's nice to see that some still pay tribute to the old-fashioned virtues of hard work". Then she wandered off and soon faded into the distance in one of the brightly lit corridors. In the coming weeks and months, I would spend several moments trying to convince Mrs Weber not to leave the building.

The receptionist thanked me for my help and escorted me to one of the meeting rooms, where I was to be joined by the home's head of care for an introductory talk. She explained that I was now in the main building. The main building boasts function rooms, the main nursing office (internally referred to as the "pool"), and some sanitary facilities for both visitors and employees. The large window front opens to a small garden park with young trees and colourful flowerbeds. The park accommodates a meandering, circular promenade, alongside an aviary and a rabbit hutch. At the heart and centre of the garden, the so-called village square offers benches from which one may witness the water play in a small, electrically operated fountain. Where the park is not marked off by one of the four houses or the main building, some green and a fence keep the residents safe. I would later learn that the entrance to the garden is designed in a way that invites residents to go for a spin. This is to ensure that residents with orientation difficulties cannot leave the terrain without proper guidance. To mirror a German village structure, two of the four houses are detached. In order to reach them, one needs to cross the park.

Matt, the head of care, entered the room. He was in his early 40s, slender, with a strong jaw. Personable yet controlled in his demeanour, he appeared to be hands-on, pragmatic and continuously on the run. Indeed, this morning it seemed as though he held the home together with little more than his phone and his calm disposition. The phone was ringing every few minutes, so he needed to leave our meeting quite regularly. When he returned, he would apologise for the disruption, whereupon he would continue to tell me about the home and that he had only recently joined the team. When we spoke, he was welcoming and sincere. He promptly revealed in no uncertain terms that he was not interested in portraying the project in only a good light, but also aimed to show me "what is really going on". On the day of our initial meeting, he was unhappy with how disorganised the home was. When I began my fieldwork, 27 residents had already moved in, amounting to half of the home's capacity.

Matt's new post was tailored to his strengths and attuned to his career trajectory:

> I'm coming from another home, and was ready for this challenge. There's so much right with this home's visions and yet still so much wrong with how we're doing things. Right now we can't provide the quality here that I had initiated in the former home I worked at. But it's hard. The foundation wants to break even and doesn't give us the staff we need.

He spoke in a conversational tone, obviously aware of everything there was still to do. "I know that you're coming from the Netherlands", he continued. "Hogewey is a great project, but they have so many more financial resources at their disposal; something like that is not possible in Germany, despite our best intentions". While he was happy with the initial concept of the home, he articulated many enhancements that needed to be addressed. He then offered to show me around.

The Brickyard Mansion

We stepped into the first of four houses, the Villa Ziegelhof ("Brickyard Mansion"). The interior was designed in a modern and contemporary style, with brightly coloured walls. Matt then took me to one of the unoccupied rooms, the "showroom", as they call it. It was spacious and, aside from one bed, there was no furniture. Matt explained: "The residents ought to bring their own furniture, in order to feel at home, that's important, you know, so they have some memorabilia. When residents move in, it leaves a void, and familiar surroundings need to fill it". The bathrooms were generous and finished from floor to ceiling with white tiles, which gave them a slightly clinical feel. They were easily accessible by wheelchair and the floors were evenly levelled. The shower was in the corner, and no doors obstructed access. All the amenities were state-of-the-art. "Do you lock the doors at night?" I asked. "No, we don't", he responded, continuing:

> You know, I believe that if we succeed in sheltering the residents from all danger, we will have failed as carers. This should not be a golden cage. It's interesting, the relatives would rather have us increase security and lock the individual doors at night. At the same time, the social romantics criticise us for having the village fenced off, so one's mother or father can't 'run there'.

I asked why he said "run there" as opposed to "run off", to which he replied: "We say danger of 'running to' [*Hinlaufgefahr*], not 'running off' [*Weglaufgefahr*], because for the residents, they don't feel that they are running away. They are going somewhere, they want to go home, or shopping, or whatever. So they are not running away". He continued to tell me about an event that had occurred recently:

> Two weeks ago we had one resident disappear. The two carers on the night shift called me. It was the weekend. They had looked everywhere, but they didn't find her. So they called me in the middle of the night and we eventually had to call the police, and they came with a helicopter. We looked everywhere in the surrounding woods. It was late at night. Eventually we found the resident in the closet of an empty room, anxious and distraught. We were lucky to find her inside the village. But you see, when you're dealing with such cases, hearing people's criticism of the fences becomes laughable. Obviously it would be nice to live in a free and happy environment, but if something happens to a resident, if they get lost, or if they drown in the lake, who will be held responsible? The same voices will ask: 'Why didn't anybody stop her?' Sometimes the dementia discourse is packed with hypocrisy.

In order for the residents to "feel" free and remain safe, the dementia village needs to draw clear boundaries. Where are the fences? How high can they be? Which doors should be locked? Which rooms ought to be accessible? How much hygiene is needed? The extent of freedom is highly negotiated between concerns for safety and freedom. On our way to the second house, we strolled by a couple sitting on the porch. I was about to introduce myself but immediately sensed the weight of the moment we were walking into. The wife was a new resident. Ever since she had moved to the village, her husband would dutifully visit her every day, generally in the afternoon. They were sitting next to each other on two wooden lawn chairs. The wife was fighting back tears. We caught snippets of the conversation: "and you always told me, no, no, you'll be back, don't worry", she said. Her husband spoke thoughtfully and deliberately, "Yes, that's what I said". The wife's voice started trembling and cracking: "And I told you that I don't want that. You don't need to care for me; I'm perfectly capable of taking care of myself. Once I go back to school, and my house, then I'm happy. You might as well have thrown me into the Weser [the local river]".

The husband looked at us, as though searching for comfort and reassurance. He then replied with casual interest, "I told you again and again, you can't come home". The wife noticed our presence and managed a tight-lipped smile. But her breathing was rapid and her face flushed with turmoil. Matt raised an eyebrow and answered his phone. We then walked across the square in the centre of the village, past the village fountain. On our way, Matt told me that the wife had repeatedly locked out her husband and called the police, whereupon her two sons and husband had decided to bring her to the home. Additionally, she suffered from Hepatitis C, which made caring for her difficult, as one constantly needed to be cautious not to get infected. "It's hard to move to a new place at this age. With emigration comes loss and then grieving". Matt let this hang in the air for a moment, then continued:

> You surely know Elisabth Kübler-Ross' (1969) work. In her five stages of grief, the first is denial. In the beginning, many residents deny that they have actually left. But as the days tick by, the permanence of the move will sink in. But this is a journey they need to take together with their loved ones. And we need the families to be involved.

Indeed, the home's management deems the families' involvement an important element in the care routine. "The fates of family members and residents", an internal care document states, "are inextricably linked". For this reason, besides their daily nursing duties, the staff are responsible for offering family members information, guidance and clarification with regard to their relatives in the home. Family members and caregivers are advised to be in close contact to understand and support each other effectively. According to the village's administration, this is achieved through several means. First, and prior to their relative's entry, the families receive information about the particular services offered in the housing communities. Second, they are asked for biographical information and memorabilia that might make it easier for the relative to settle in and feel at home in the new environment. Third, the family ideally provides comprehensive information on the relative's possible behavioural problems, their background, their household routines and potential issues that may arise. Fourth, the families are encouraged to be involved in everyday nursing routines and the care design. Should a resident be dissatisfied, their family will be approached early and it will be stressed that all criticism will be perceived as an incentive to improve care and not as a personal attack. This is ideally facilitated through regular family events and a dialogue with the carers.

The Lakeside Mansion

We moved to the next house, the Villa am See ("Lakeside Mansion"), the décor of which, according to the prospectus, was classic and timeless. The walls were painted in warm red and brown colours. Here, all residents had already moved in. The houses were connected through a glass hallway, something Matt was not happy about. "The initial idea really was that the houses stand individually and not connected, but well, we haven't fully managed to have this materialised. Safety and comfort had to come first". We walked through the sitting room, past a TV area with a giant state-of-the-art television, several sofas, and a bookcase filled with the works of many famous poets and authors, fairy tales and children's books. On the bottom shelf, I saw various board games and play materials—the sort one finds in typical German households, ranging from *Mensch Ärgere Dich Nicht* (Ludo), checkers and playing cards to a myriad of colourful jigsaw puzzles and two large foam dice.

Most of the residents had already eaten and were either relaxing in their rooms or taking a rest on the sun terrace. On the terrace, six women were sitting around a wooden table, serenely drinking coffee and water and looking out upon the neat flower beds and the village's pastoral peace. To protect the residents from the harsh, unyielding sunlight, a dark blue parasol had been stretched to cover. The ladies sat in silence with a seeming calmness about their twilight years. Every now and then one would utter a brief comment, either about a carer passing by, the heat or the bees and flies that kept settling upon every brightly coloured piece of clothing. In the background, one could hear the gardener mowing the terraced lawn behind the building; a smell of freshly cut grass and petrol from the mower lingered in the air. Beside the table, several wheeled walkers were parked together. An elegantly dressed woman in her early 60s, with bleached blond teased hair, was trying to cut through the convoluted line of walkers. She wanted to retire to her room and shot us a nervous glance. Matt tended to her well-being and wished her a good rest. Then a prim-looking carer walked out of the house, carrying more glasses. "Let's make sure we all drink lots of water, we need it in this heat", she said cheerfully, while pouring glasses of water for everyone.

The Ridingyard Mansion

We returned inside the house and walked down a bright, glass façade corridor that connected the Villa am See with the third mansion, the Villa Reithof ("Ridingyard Mansion"). This third edifice overlooked the horse stables next door. The stables formed a striking contrast to the newly built care village. The grass needed cutting, the roof patching, and quite a few surfaces warranted a fresh coat of paint. The décor of the mansion was in the style of a country home. Matt then led me into the dining area, which was separated from the kitchen by a countertop, cluttered with leftovers from lunch. A feisty young carer with long dark hair was brushing off bits of salad and pasta from dishes and utensils before loading them into the dishwasher. Eight tables with chairs were arranged alongside the window front. Meanwhile, two residents were finishing their desserts in the dining area. One resident was singing the same verse of an old German children's song. Every now and then the carer would sing along with the resident by starting a new verse. The singing resident then made a violent lunge for her table neighbour's spoon and began tapping on the wooden table. By the look on her neighbour's face, this created an unsettling sound. The neighbour then stood up, rambled a bit, and dashed off to her room. Nearer to the carer, another resident was casually leaning against the counter, overlooking the kitchen. There seemed to be a warm quiet between the two. The carer would steal cheeky glances at the resident, and the resident would smile back. Yet due to the neighbouring horses and the summer heat, the carers struggled to cope with the flies sneaking into the house. One carer, folding clothes, was frantically killing the insects with a fly swatter. "This is the home I'd prefer for myself", Matt declared. "You see the horses from the window, so there's always something going on".

The home's care philosophy posits that the staff see the residents' behavioural syndromes as expressions of self-help, self-preservation and self-protection. Their actions are understood as a response to the feeling of loss that the residents experience. Also, any abnormal behaviour from a resident is appreciated as the resident's way of adjusting to their new realities and compensating for their shortfall in other communicative means. In that vein, challenging behaviour is recognised as a self-healing attempt in response to physical, mental or social wounds incurred as a result of the disease. The behaviour is thus not perceived as a deficit, but triggered by the deeply painful losses and interventions in the residents' lives.

Consequently, the carers are encouraged to see challenging behavioural manifestations as residents' subjective and meaningful engagement with their own bereavement. Instead of surpassing the symptoms of such self-help attempts, the carers are meant to connect with each resident, to discuss, and to strive to understand the individual's loss. Reportedly, there is a wide range of behavioural symptoms. While the residents frequently undergo a personality change, their emotional feeling (it is stressed) is not clouded and their ability to direct attention to external stimuli remains. With this understanding of behavioural problems in mind, the carers are believed to be more successful in empathising with the residents. For the latter, the experience of distance and proximity is sometimes skewed. While potentially incomprehensible to an outsider, residents often seek close body contact to get attention, to make themselves heard, or to deal with stressful circumstances. Furthermore, fear and distrust—and even hallucinations or delusions—may occur and unpremeditated, new or unpleasant situations such as a visit to the hairdressers or the doctor may cause fear and distress. Internal tensions and torment can lead to excessive motor activity, even agitation. Restlessness and confusion may increase in the evenings, which is referred to as "sun downing" and is often accompanied by a strong inclination to run away, or, in adapted care speech, to "run to". Conversely, a lack of drive and motivation can occur, paired with a higher perception and expression of pain. Lastly, feelings of hunger and thirst generally decrease, and, sooner or later, the residents ordinarily become incontinent.

The Hastebach Mansion

The last house we visited was the Villa Hastebach ("Hasty Brook Mansion"), which was named after the small stream meandering through the countryside not far from the house. With blue and white walls, giving it a Nordic Scandinavian feel, the mansion was still uninhabited. Some carers had cut out a few paper fish for decoration, some of which were already dangling from the roof. Next door, the former brickyard was being rebuilt into a day-care centre. "The idea is that the residents will be able to join some of their activities once it's finished", Matt declared. "This ought to offer them some more activities, while at the same time relieve the carers in the village. In general, there is no forced sociability". He continued: "If residents want to spend the evening with other residents, it should be because they really want to".

After taking a slight detour around the ward, we once again crossed the village square to return to Matt's office. On our way we encountered another resident. She was sitting in one of the flowerbeds, engrossed in playing with some stones, watching the dirt slip through her fingers. As we passed, she noticed us. She stood up, gingerly brushing the dirt off her trousers and moving a strand of her silver hair out of her face. With one foot bare and the other wearing a wet sock, she stood rooted to the spot. Her tan highlighted her finely chiselled features, emphasising the magnetic quality of her clear green eyes. Matt introduced me to her, mentioning that she had previously been a yoga teacher. She gave me an amicable smile. With a natural dignity and presence, she reached out her hand and placed it on my arm. "How wonderful to finally meet you", she said enthusiastically. "It's quite warm, isn't it. Yes, it is indeed. And the flowers are just blooming like there's no tomorrow, it's just marvellous". I agreed and asked her if the hot weather was not bothering her. She looked at the sky, then away from it and back at it again. She then shut her eyes as though she were squeezing out a thought. She pointed at some tiny clouds in the sky and said, "I see it coming already, you know, these big, big, you know… you never know what's going to happen, life is full of surprises, isn't it?" I asked her if she enjoyed living in the home. She replied: "Oh, there's always a little of this and that. You never stop learning, isn't that so? And this here [pointing to the bush behind her], it's quite remarkable, quite remarkable I tell you. But I think I had better get back to work now". We said goodbye and she returned to her spot and resumed digging up stones. Mrs Edwards, Matt informed me, had been brought to the home by her son, a famous heart surgeon from the north of Germany. She had gone missing for several days in the city before someone eventually discovered her in a garden shed. What was remarkable about our conversation was that Mrs Edwards seemed to formulate well thought-out and coherent sentences, at normal volume and speed and with a conversational tone. Her speech was nevertheless detached from reality and context, just as her behaviour and attire did not really match the conduct normally associated with that of an elderly, elegant woman. "In a regular nursing home, Mrs Edwards probably wouldn't be allowed to dress like that or play with dirt", Matt told me while we walked back to his office. "But we don't presume to know what she wants and enjoys, we provide a safe, familiar and human environment, so she can do what she enjoys. They don't come here to die, but to live".

Discussion

When the village was inaugurated in March 2014, the project's chief administrator did not mince her words: "Here we see how care work works in the 21st century. This is a great project for Hamelin, it is a great day for the city". And the chairwoman of the Tönebön foundation added, with reference to the village's critics, that the residents should not be seen as having been "deported" or "marginalised", as they would continue to partake in Hamelin's social life. "We want to make their daily routine as normal as possible", she emphasised, maintaining that what and where they eat is up to the residents themselves. "The refrigerator door is open to anyone, anytime. If someone wants to make coffee in the morning or eat a yoghurt, they can". The village is a primary example of "full in-patient care where the residents remain self-determined", which is "very labour intensive" (Keller 2014).[17]

The home had two advantages when it opened its doors. First, it could model its design and principles on the successfully implemented Dutch care home, learning from the Dutch experience and continuing the tried and tested approach. This circumstance proved vital in convincing investors and critics. Second, the model's novelty and progressive methods invited not only many families and individuals from around Germany to consider it as a potential care home, but equally grabbed the interest of many carers.[18] A few weeks after the inaugural celebrations, when I first visited, the village was still in turmoil. Undertaking a new project and implementing new processes is always a bumpy road, and launching the first German dementia village proved no exception. When I began my fieldwork, the care staff comprised 18 team members (15 women, 3 men), and the residents occupied two of the four houses, with more residents moving in every day. Management did not know how much staff was needed, who exactly would move in, or how things would work in detail. The residents had been uprooted from their former lives, the new workers needed to acclimatise to their new environment, and all of this occurred in the presence of much uncertainty. In between the intricate rules and philosophies laid out in the village's blueprint, and the frantic everyday care routine, there often was not much space for contemplation. Before we thus venture deeper into the everyday care routine, it is worthwhile to bring more attention to the idea of a dementia village.

Gemeinschaft und Gesellschaft (Community and Society)

The dementia village, by its very concept and application, creates a new demarcated space for its residents governed by societal standards of care. The residents live in the community. The carers, on the other hand, fulfil a societal function. They come in from outside to work, but do not live with the residents. This distinction between the two concepts—community on the one hand and society on the other—ties into a long-standing tradition in social thought that speaks to the tension of combining sociality with rationalised bureaucratic efficiency. Ferdinand Tönnies (2001) distinguished this as a tension between *Gemeinschaft* and *Gesellschaft*.

The concepts of *Gemeinschaft* and *Gesellschaft*, Tönnies (2001, pp. 27 f.; p. 254) argued, form the ideal types of social organisation. *Gemeinschaft* represents the communal society, in which personal relationships are structured based on time-honoured social rules. Tönnies differentiated between three original types of community, bound together by blood, proximity or conscious thought, which he referred to as kinship, neighbourhood and friendship/comradeship. Each of these forms of community is defined by a specific set of roles and a distinct awareness of the place each person occupies in the group. The members' worth and status stems from knowing who they are, where they come from and where they belong. Their worth is not tied to their achievements. This, however, also implies immobility, in both physical and social terms. Members commonly stay in one place and remain in their hierarchical positions. What follows is that a community is, by its very nature, exclusive. People outside the community may be welcomed as guests or workers who provide services on a temporary or permanent basis. They might even, with time and commitment, become passive members. Yet they hardly ever take on the role of a representative. Exclusion, not inclusion, characterises the communal spirit. While solidarity is at its core, it is also the core of a clearly defined circle, the borders of which are difficult to cross.

In contrast to the concept of community, Tönnies' notion of *Gesellschaft* embodies an association that is regulated by modern, multicultural societies with their governmental bureaucracies and sizable institutions. Society comprises individuals who may coexist peacefully but are, in essence, substantially separated. In this manner, it is every man for himself, living in a perpetual state of tension. The union is characterised by reciprocity, wherein for every service rendered and good provided, a return is not only expected but legally and socially required. In these social relations, roles are soluble and fluid, and individuals are detached from one another and become separate selves in the same way that deeds and goods become separate entities. "In *Gemeinschaft*", Tönnies (2001, p. 52) writes, "[people] stay together in spite of everything that separates them, in *Gesellschaft* they remain separate in spite of everything that unites them".[19]

In the dementia village, there is a contrast between the residents and the carers as of the village. The reality of living in a specially designed village is that it makes reality feel just that little bit less real at times. Whereas the home was designed to be a "village" in which carers would cook with patients, do laundry with them, and so on—a village in which everything would resemble civic life—there is evidently a division into groups. Most prominently, residents and carers do not form part of a community existing side by side, but have very different interests and roles. For the carers, it is a job, but also a calling. And the residents form, similar to any other "village", an inherently diverse and dynamic group. Some are happy and thankful, others are aggressive, hitting and punching the carers, and others are sad and depressed. If you take a group of people and put them in a village, naturally you will find quite a wide variety of hobbies, sleep patterns, food preferences and so on. To build a community in Tönnies' truest sense of *Gemeinschaft*, a care village, one could argue, ought to evolve internally; it should not be an organisation representing a form of *Gesellschaft*, driven by a single overbearing vision.

When thinking about the dementia village, we thus need to reflect on the often unasked and unanswered questions with which we need to reckon in a discourse about dementia care. As we have seen, several key themes ran through the media reports on the village, and the idea of a dementia village seemed to take on a life of its own. A tenaciously repeated opinion posited the concept of normality as the foundation of the care village. But what is normality? And if we need a care home to feign it, what is wrong with normality outside the confines of an institution? The principle of normality is, of course, an entirely subjective matter and defining it involves a normative, culturally informed choice. In order to exist within an institution, the care home must necessarily dictate how normality ought to be experienced and lived, because otherwise order and safety could be threatened. If one resident's idea of normality includes singing at midnight, another's normal sleep pattern might be disturbed. The recourse to normality thus entails a moral and even political evaluation by which the cohabitation form is mediated. For this reason, the concept of normality is, in each instance, a debatable principle.[20]

One of the striking differences between the German and Dutch model concerns the idea of community building within the village—or how normality is conceived. The Dutch village created different life worlds for their residents, wherein the residents' backgrounds and former habits formed the basis of their cohabitation groups. In Germany, this approach was not adopted. On the contrary, the idea was rejected—possibly due to the nation's very sensitive history with segregation and the idea of health care being distributed equally. The shared commonality of the residents, besides the fact that they were all German citizens, was their need for care. One of the project's initiators phrased it as follows:

> Whereas in Amsterdam the houses are divided amongst different groups of patients, according to their hobbies and origins, we didn't copy this aspect of their model. Here we have rural communities, people share similar origins, and their houses are not divided. You may find a former sales assistant, a teacher, and, yes, even a professor might move in. And we didn't differentiate between those groups.

Another carer was a bit more blunt, saying: "Can you imagine? Separating people based on background in Germany? We might as well call it the Third Reich village!" An administrator, in turn, stressed that there is no singular admission criterion that exhausts the possibilities of the concept. Rather, the village concept should always be situated within particular contexts:

> If we had followed the idea of the dementia village to the letter, this would beg the question of how demented you need to be to be admitted to the village. And I know of families who'd rather take their mother or father to a local care home that does not specialise in dementia, as otherwise everyone would immediately think she is mad. So there is still a lot of educa-

> tional work ahead in order for the condition not be as disreputable. I think that whether you physically or mentally depend on care, there shouldn't be a difference.

These social differences could lead to friction with those residents who did not feel at home amongst the other residents. The exclusionary principle of the Dutch dementia village collided with the German understanding of equal health care provision. Certainly, the initiators of Hamelin's dementia village never strived to create an exact replica of the Dutch dementia village. They explicitly adopted a "mix and match" strategy for the project, to the extent that the carers often yearned for more structure than the model was initially designed for—a structure that would categorise residents according to the degree of their dementia progression in order for them to fulfil their professional duties better. The differences in the way in which the Dutch and German dementia villages conceived and delivered their care services does not mean that one approach is right and the other is wrong, or that one necessarily offers more person-centred or individual care. It only means that they are different, and that certain socio-cultural values inherent in the existing arrangements probably come into play.

By its very nature, an ethnographic account cannot demonstrate either the generalisability or predictive power claimed by other scientific disciplines, which tend to approximate such ideals more closely than ethnography can, ever will and indeed should. Then again, ethnography derives its efficacy in no small measure from the insight that there are limits to our interpretations. It builds its strength by knowing its boundaries. This paper does therefore not depict an entire country or culture or a token programme representing Germany in a strong and distinctive fashion on a macro level. While it is vital to allow for both cultural and environmental factors (Jacobson 1991), we should refrain from artificially establishing national binaries.[21] Nevertheless, by pointing out the difference between the Dutch and German model, we can see how they both grew from deep historical and ideological roots. The same is the case with Tönnies' conception of *Gemeinschaft*. Whereas his evaluation is structured around a sequence of conceptual dualistic contraries—or what he called "normal types"—they are not merely abstract analytical tools.[22] In

Tönnies' (2001, p. 17) view, social relations may be understood either as originating from genuine, natural bonds, which are the heart and soul of communities, or as an essentially mechanistic formation, steeped in reason and thought, which is what we conceive of as a society. This differentiation evidently implies certain judgements. Indeed, Tönnies framed his normal types with the underlying notion that naturally evolved social relationships in the community are favourable. By contrast, artificial and systematic relations in society are "predatory and pathological, a distinction that [bears] all the hallmarks, not of the 'mechanistic' outlook of the scientific enlightenment, but of Aristotelian and medieval scholastic roots" (2001, p. xxvii). The straightforward division between community and society does not conceal the circumstance that defining and using a community as an empirical field of study is a tricky and controversial task. "In considering the concept of community", Colin Bell and Howard Newby (1971, p. 2) maintain, "the sociologist shares an occupational hazard with the architect and the planner; the more he attempts to define it in his own terms, the more elusive does the essence of it seem to escape him". Too often, subjective value judgments colour the description of a community, and the mere definition of a group as a community might—and indeed often does—involve one's normative recommendation of what it should be.[23] Just as the conceptual notion of "contract" dominated the intellectual discourse throughout the Age of Reason, "community" occupied a powerful position in the attitudes of nineteenth century sociological thinkers. The concept was not merely a callous, methodical instrument for reaching an empirical description of social relationships. Rather, the term accompanied an undercurrent of positive and nostalgic associations, to the extent that the move from close personal and communal bonds to the contractual, utilitarian and impersonal relations found in an emerging industrial society was often lamented (Bell and Newby 1971).

Comte, for instance, held that Western states had emerged out of political and industrial revolutions and were abnormal and artificial fabrications, both dangerous and lacking emotional and social competence. He feared that modern-day authorities were negligent in taking care of their population. In view of the vast diversity in the populace and to regain a sense of community and connection, he suggested that modern states be broken down into smaller units, comprising cities, towns and their surrounding countryside (Pickering 2009). In *Suicide*, Emile Durkheim (1897) expressed concern that the decay of collective conscience and the deterministic shift to individualism was causing the fall of long-established communities. This could lead to what he termed "anomie", or a complete and utter loss of societal norms. Yet, as opposed to Comte, he believed that the rising division of labour would, while destroying traditional communal ties, lead to the formation of new and bigger organic communities, as different types of solidarity would emerge.

Lastly, Karl Marx's use of the term "community" exemplifies the contrast in usage that pervades the above thinkers' accounts. On the one hand, Marx held a more descriptive sense of the concept and saw community as a group of people living together as a collective and sharing various historical, social and economic ties. These primitive communities, which he refers to as "natural communities", stand in contrast to the feudal community that, for centuries, formed the backbone of medieval European society. On the other hand, Marx held a normative prescription of community, which he would sometimes term "the real community". This represented Marx's notion of freedom, wherein one does not depend on the servitude of others (Brenkert 1983). Tönnies indeed demonstrated his affinity to many Marxian notions of capitalism throughout his work and applied several elements of Marx's ideas to his conceptual framework. Ultimately, however, he understood the emergence of a trade-heavy capitalistic society not so much as a cause for the demise of community, but turned Marx's thesis around and argued for a structural explanation. In this fashion, he claimed that the loss of communal life provided a fertile ground for the growth of new social organisations (Cahnman 1973). Irrespective of their diverse approaches, all these accounts share a certain praise and positive regard for community. They see in it "man's natural habitat" (Bell and Newby 1971, p. 22), endangered by the faceless, impersonal and anonymous industrial society. A strong sense of nostalgia and an unsettling sense of placelessness accompany most thinkers' images of fading communal life. In the words of Keith Melville (1972, p. 171), however:

> The danger of any form of nostalgia is that it is so simple to imagine a past which never existed. It is seductively easy to assume that, until the

> beginning of the industrial age, community universally mean that one was always close to the warm bosom of cherished friends and welcome traditions.

Tönnies' theory provides a simplistic notion of community and society. Implementing one automatically rules out the other. In the real historical world, however, the two types coexist; the boundaries are permeable. The dementia village presents a case in point. For that reason, it is not a question of whether individuals and organisations, in their thoughts and actions, form exclusively a *Gemeinschaft* or *Gesellschaft*. Rather, the question is where on the spectrum between these two poles the object of enquiry is located (Tönnies 2001, p. xxviii). We must bear this in mind when further exploring the village's notions of community and society. While it is tempting to recognise the two concepts as physical, tangible bodies, the very character of a social group does not lie in its biological or geographical qualities but in the inherent relational connections that bind the group together.[24]

Conclusion

"A brain is a terrible thing to watch waste away", uttered the amateur gardener of the labyrinthine allotment gardens when I asked her for directions to the new dementia village. Her remark called up an image of a rotting brain that had once ripened. As some accounts in this paper have illustrated, however, life in a dementia care home can be much better than what is suggested in some of the mortifying clinical portrayals. Questions addressing appropriate and novel ideas for dementia care, however, also resonate in utopian and theoretical accounts of community, of which the dementia village is an example. The longing for more inclusive, collective care models that emphasise human relationships and solidarity rather than calculated self-interest is found in many care circles. It is felt as profoundly as the discontent with the diminishing bonds of kinship and family seen in nineteenth century thought. Yet the universality of home—or, in this particular case, "the village" as a place for care—leads us to comprehend it as both undisputed and natural, and we tend to neglect or underrate the ways in which it is culturally determined.

Such ideas are strengthened by the common yet precarious view of home and community as the "natural" place of care and effortless relationships that are bound by emotions and connection, while medicine and cure carry the connotation of knowledge and comprehension of facts. The dementia village project evolved amongst many human and touching experiences, thankful relatives, husbands visiting their wives every day and a strong team spirit and cohesion amongst the carers.[25] The home, designed to be a village in which everything resembles civic life, might not have met this vision, but it did not lack humanity. It did not lack care. Neither did I encounter insufficient or bad care. The carers did care, and most of them with sensitivity, rather than sentimentality. Nonetheless, the rising prevalence of chronic illnesses means that care is becoming an increasingly complex affair. It is with due regard for these actualities that we must construe the relationships between the village residents, the carers, dementia and social life. And I hope that by outlining some of these complexities, this paper will foster a deeper and more critical understanding of dementia, ageing and the care we all hope to receive in our twilight years.

Notes

1. In the mid-1960s, social psychologist Richard Kalish (1966) introduced the notion of "psychological death", referring to a demise of consciousness resulting in the individual ceasing to be aware of their own self. Thus, the individual not only forgets *who* they are but also *that* they are. Arthur Kleinman (1988), in turn, forcefully argued that language and social exclusion, consciously or unconsciously, can lead to a descent into a passive solitude, which literally engenders "social death" (also see George 2010).
2. The impaired ability to both learn new information (working memory) and recall previously learned information (long-term memory) (Weiner and Lipton 2009, p. 47).
3. Language disturbance (Weiner and Lipton 2009, p. 47).
4. The inability to carry out motor activities in spite of intact motor function (e.g. strength and coordination) (Weiner and Lipton 2009, p. 47).
5. A failure to either recognise or identify objects in spite of intact sensory function (Weiner and Lipton 2009, p. 47).

6. For instance, planning, organising, sequencing or abstracting (Weiner and Lipton 2009, p. 47).
7. See, for instance, Townsend 1952; Goffman 1961; Foucault 1989 (1963); Zola 1972; Rosenhan 1973; Smith 1974; Noddings 1984; Gubrium 1986; or Weinberg 2005.
8. Branded as an innovative, humane and affordable model of dementia care, the village today hosts around 150 residents, averaging 83 years of age. Roughly 250 full- and part-time health care workers and local volunteers care for the residents. The residents live in 23 different homes, each catering for 6 or 7 residents. These are categorised in seven diverse "lifestyle categories", which entail housing for the Dutch upper class, homemakers, trade/craftsmen and women as well as religious, cultured, Indonesian (for those who most value their ethnic heritage) or urban residents. Two core principles govern the village. First, the village strives to give residents a home in which they are surrounded by recognisable objects and people with similar values, backgrounds and interests, in order to create experiences that are reminiscent of the resident's formative years. Second, much emphasis is placed on keeping the residents active and in a safe environment. Twenty-five clubs offer activities that include folksong, bingo, painting, cycling, literature and baking (Zorggroep (2016); Berry 2013; Carpenter (2012); Henley 2012; Tagliabue 2012).
9. See, for instance, Grün 1998; Hurley 2012; Jenkins and Smythe 2013; or Hogewoning-van der Vossen 2004.
10. In Switzerland, a care centre in the form of a mock-1950s is currently under construction, intended to cater exclusively to elderly residents with Alzheimer's and other dementias (Grogg 2014; Paterson 2012). In the UK, a replica village high street was recently built at a dementia care home in Suffolk to help the residents retrieve some of their memories (BBC 2014). Also see Keller (2013) for other German projects.
11. The 650 hours correspond with the carers' work schedule. I generally conducted participant observations during entire work shifts. Nightshifts would usually last up to 11 hours, whereas dayshifts spanned over a period of 8 hours. I did not explicitly call the interviews such; they were often down-to-earth chats peppered with banter, confessions and life stories. As the later chapters will illustrate, they were far from formal. They took place in between and on the way, over coffee and during cigarette breaks, on benches and table chairs and while peeling potatoes or washing up, brushing someone's hair, cleaning the floors, consoling a crying resident or chuckling over a joke while pulling support stockings over someone's feet. The open-endedness of ethnography offers this

much-needed flexibility, making it, in the words of Sarah Franklin and Celia Roberts (2006, p. 93), "radically exploratory". Initially, valuable findings took the form of questions, rather than answers.

12. In order to bring more clarity by way of a culturally informed view of dementia, I took a position—one also adopted by anthropologists Margaret Lock (1993, 2002) and Tsipy Ivry (2010)—that understands knowledge about our bodies and minds as a product of history and culture. When addressing the mythologies of menopause in Japan and North America, Lock (1993, p. 370) pithily concluded that the condition "is neither fact nor universal event but an experience that we must interpret in context". To quote Darin Weinberg (2005, p. 7), "social studies of science have shown time and again that scientific discoveries are temporally situated social constructions rather than revelations of a timeless and uniform natural order". In this view, care practices stem from their "embeddedness" in systems and ideas about health and illness, individuality and selfhood that exist in a "productive network" that permeates the social body in its entirety (Foucault 1980, p. 243).
13. In the English-speaking world, the tale is primarily known for Robert Browning's poem *The Pied Piper of Hamelin* (Curren et al. 1942).
14. Perhaps the greatest ironic juxtaposition, however, is that Hamelin is also home to Germany's largest juvenile detention centre, which lies less than 1 km south of the newly built village. Hamelin's youth detention centre provides accommodation for young people between the ages of 14 and 24 who are remanded in custody or sentenced to a period of confinement, of which the average length is 1.7 years. Although it didn't open its doors until 1980, Hamelin's prison history goes back a long way. It dates back to the Thirty Years' War (1618–1648), after which Hamelin was converted into a large country fortress. As such, it served as a prison for the "dangerous subjects of the country". Throughout the following centuries, new buildings were added and the prison was continuously expanded. During the Nazi dictatorship, it was used to detain political prisons, opponents of the regime and homosexuals (40 of whom were violently liquidated in April 1945). In the post-war years, the British government briefly used it as a detention centre for war criminals and added an execution site. Once returned to the federal state of Niedersachsen (in 1950), it was eventually converted into a juvenile detention centre. The 150-year-old prison, however, proved entirely unsuitable as a juvenile prison, which is why a new building was erected in the south of the city (Jugendanstalt Hameln 2015).

15. The sections discussing the home's care philosophy are primarily based on extensive interviews with the head of care and manager of the village, as well as internal documents and guidelines to which I was given access.
16. To protect her identity and the identities of all other residents and carers discussed in this paper, I have observed the convention of changing the name and defining characteristics.
17. The vision of full in-patient care in which residents remain self-determined inaugurates a thematic dimension of this paper—namely, understanding dementia care as a way of managing contradictory and complex demands for safety, health and autonomy.
18. When I began my fieldwork, several hundred carers had already sent in their applications, some frustrated with the bureaucratic and rigid work environments in other establishments, some inspired by the concept's apparent uniqueness, and others displeased with other homes' prevalent tendency to medicate residents.
19. At the time, Tönnies' assertions and theories contested widely held views of German philosophical circles. He challenged the then distinct tendency in late nineteenth century political thought to overly confine itself to the "individualism vs. collectivism" debate. Tönnies claimed that drawing a clear line between the two concepts was a futile endeavour, as both simply embody two separate forms of individualism (Merz-Benz 1991; Walther 1991).
20. Without a doubt, psychological and sociological literature, alone, is replete with examples of discussions of "normality". To name but two: Margaret Lock (2013, p. 42) engages in detail with the biomedical side of dementia research and includes a detailed discussion of the relationship between dementia and normal ageing. Drawing on Michel Foucault and Auguste Comte's work, she writes that "until well into the 19th century use of the term 'normal' was virtually limited to the fields of mathematics and physics. It was not until an internalising approach to the body based on anatomy took hold that arguments about the relationship between normal and abnormal biological states were seriously debated for the first time". In *Concepts of Normality: The Autistic and Typical Spectrum* (2008), Wendy Lawson, on the other hand, compellingly outlines theories behind the Western conception that has led to a culture that fails to be inclusive.
21. Nevertheless, my research reveals levels of explanation that touch on national or cultural idiosyncrasies in the observed care approach. Such differences include political-economic variances, contrary ideas of

autonomy and family ethics, and contrasting gendered expectations. Yet, as George Marcus and Dick Cushman (1982, p. 31) note, traditional chapters on "geography, kinship, economics, politics and religion" merely suggest the theoretical stance that societies can be synthetically divided into such analytical elements.

22. Tönnies wrote his influential work at a time when the German empire was striving for national unity, ready to take great leaps forward to achieve their lofty goals. In 1878, when the first edition of *Gemeinschaft und Gesellschaft* was published, the German election had been won by the Conservatives, while the Liberals and Social Democrats had lost many seats. National unity was not achieved as a result of a republican movement, as had happened in neighbouring France, or as a compromise between the democratic bourgeoisie with the nobility in England. Rather, unity was the result of an imperial alliance of German states under the hegemony of the Prussian nobility. Germany was missing the embourgeoisement that had taken place in England, the Netherlands and America. Seven years before, the young state had won the Franco-German War and the resulting tribute payments from France boosted German industry. Meanwhile, with the onset of industrialisation, emerging cries for social change began to undermine the once resilient feudal order, which spurred on a strong and confident labour movement. These new influences found themselves facing the old forces of nobility, the Church and the politically weak bourgeoisie. While Tönnies sympathised with the labour movement, he did not necessarily see his role in advancing the processes fuelled by socialist theory. Rather, he wanted to enhance the civil structures needed to achieve a democratic-republican civility. It was this contract for civility that he attempted to fulfil in his function as a social scientist, and he did so by juxtaposing the social philosophy of the contemporary German Wilhelmism and the historical school of relationalism with its roots in seventeenth century natural law. With imperial Germany lacking a sovereign rationality theory, Tönnies sought his role models in countries where reflections on civility (Hobbes in England and Spinoza in the Netherlands) had prospered more than in his native land (Merz-Benz 1991; Walther 1991).
23. They further state, "the task that faces the sociologist of the community is to generalize, whilst avoiding normative prescription, from the basis of empirical descriptions based on a myriad of theoretical positions which vary enormously in their explicitness. The studies themselves are too often incomplete descriptions of the locality because the 'problem' or the

'theory' dictated that only certain areas were investigated. This is an enormously difficult and challenging task" (1971, p. 252).

24. It must be added that whenever Tönnies addressed the purpose of communal social norms, he tended to employ historically narrow ideologies. In his view, the patriarchal form of community is the necessary consequence of evolution and is thus, by implication, the general and most natural form of community. In truth, however, this is not a mandatory result of the anthropological process but rather plays into the common myth of community as a patriarchal system. It may be the uncritical acceptance of such historical prejudices that motivated numerous political groups after the 1920s to use Tönnies' work to legitimise their conservative ideologies of community (Walther 1991).
25. It also must be noted here that care at a distance, whether physical, geographical, emotional or technological, need not result in less intensive care for patients or residents. In *Care at a Distance: On the Closeness of Technology*, for instance, Jeannette Pols (2012) persuasively demonstrates by drawing on ethnographic observations of both carers and patients involved in telecare, that there is a rise in the frequency of contact between the two.

References

Ballard, C., & Bannister, C. (2010). Criteria for the Diagnosis of Dementia. In J. O'Brian, D. Amesn, & A. Burns (Eds.), *Dementia* (pp. 31–47). London: Martin Dunitz.

BBC. (2014). Suffolk Replica Village Boosts Dementia Patient Memories. *Bbc.co.uk*. Retrieved March 3, 2016, from http://www.bbc.co.uk/news/uk-england-suffolk-28061574

Bell, C., & Newby, H. (1971). *Community Studies: An Introduction to the Sociology of the Local Community*. London: Allen and Unwin.

Berry, L. (2013). Lessons from Abroad. *Nursing Older People, 25*(6), 3.

Brenkert, G. G. (1983). *Marx's Ethics of Freedom*. Oxon: Routledge.

Cahnman, W. J. (1973). *Ferdinand Tönnies: A New Evaluation*. Leiden: E.J. Brill.

Carpenter, J. (2012). Inside Dementiaville. *Express.co.uk*. Retrieved January 31, 2016, from http://www.express.co.uk/news/retirement/299377/Inside-Dementiaville

Curren Hamm, A., & Browning, R. (1942). *Robert Browning's Pied Piper of Hamelin*. London: Tower Press.

Durkheim, E. (1951 [1897]). *Suicide*. Glencoe: Free Press.

Focus. (2012). Die Besten Pflegeheime. *FOCUS-Spezial – Wohnen & Leben im Alter, 11/12*, 56–61.

Foucault, M. (1980). *Power/Knowledge: Selected Interviews and Other Writings, 1972–1977*. Brighton: Harvester Press.

Foucault, M. (1989 [1963]). *The Birth of the Clinic—An Archaeology of Medical Perception*. Abingdon: Routledge.

Franklin, S., & Roberts, C. (2006). *Born and Made: An Ethnography of Preimplantation Genetic Diagnosis*. Oxford: Princeton University Press.

George, D. R. (2010). The Art of Medicine Overcoming the Social Death of Dementia Through Language. *The Lancet, 376*, 586–587.

Goffman, E. (1961). *Asylums: Essays on the Social Situation of Mental Patients and Other Inmates*. New York: Anchor Books.

Grogg, R. (2014). Für das Demenzdorf wird geübt. *Bernerzeitung.ch*. Retrieved March 3, 2016, from http://www.bernerzeitung.ch/region/emmental/Fuer-das-Demenzdorf-wird-geuebt/story/14390483

Grün, O. (1998). Zukünftige Organisationsstrukturen für Alters- und Pflegeheime. *Zeitschrift für Gerontologie und Geriatrie, 31*(6), 398–406.

Gubrium, J. (1986). *Oldtimers and Alzheimer's: The Descriptive Organization of Senility*. London: JAI Press Inc.

Haeusermann, T. (2017). The Dementias–A Review and a Call for a Disaggregated Approach. *Journal of Aging Studies, 42*, 22–31.

Henley, J. (2012). The Village Where People Have Dementia—And Fun. *Theguardian.com*. Retrieved March 3, 2016, from http://www.theguardian.com/society/2012/aug/27/dementia-village-residents-have-fun

Hogewoning-van der Vossen, A. (2004). Living in Lifestyle Groups in Nursing Home—Changeover to a Psychosocial Model of Care-Giving in Dementia. In G. N. M. Jones & B. M. L. Miesen (Eds.), *Care-Giving in Dementia: Research and Applications* (pp. 97–122). Hove: Brunner-Routledge.

Hurley, D. (2012). "Village of the Demented" Draws Praise as New Care Model. *Neurology Today, 12*(10), 12–13.

Ivry, T. (2010). *Embodying Culture: Pregnancy in Japan and Israel*. New Brunswick: Rutgers University Press.

Jacobson, D. (1991). *Reading Ethnography*. New York: State University of New York Press.

Jenkins, C., & Smythe, A. (2013). Reflections on a Visit to a Dementia Care Village. *Nursing Older People, 25*, 14–19.

Jugendanstalt Hameln. (2015). Herzlich Willkommen auf der Homepage der Jugendanstalt Hameln. Retrieved March 3, 2016, from http://www.

jugendanstalt-hameln.niedersachsen.de/portal/live.php?navigation_id=24052&_psmand=180

Kalish, R. A. (1966). A Continuum of Subjectively Perceived Death. *The Gerontologist, 6*(2), 73–76.

Keller, A. (2013). Demenzdorf Alzey in der Prüfung: Ist das Modell ein Pflegeheim? *News.wohnen-im-alter.de.* Retrieved March 3, 2016, from http://news.wohnen-im-alter.de/2013/07/demenzdorf-alzey-in-der-prufung-ist-das-modell-ein-pflegeheim/

Keller, A. (2014). Tönebön am See: Erstes „Demenzdorf" Deutschlands in Hameln eröffnet. *News.wohnen-im-alter.de.* Retrieved March 3, 2016, from http://news.wohnen-im-alter.de/2014/04/erstes-demenzdorf-deutschlands-hameln-eroeffnet/

Kleinman, A. (1988). *The Illness Narratives – Suffering, Healing, and the Human Condition.* New York: Basic Books.

Kübler-Ross, E. (1969). *On Death and Dying.* London: Routledge.

Lawson, W. (2008). *Concepts of Normality: The Autistic and Typical Spectrum.* London: Jessica Kingsley Publishers.

Lock, M. (1993). *Encounters with Aging: Mythologies of Menopause in Japan and North America.* London: University of California Press.

Lock, M. (2013). *The Alzheimer Conundrum: Entanglements of Dementia and Aging.* Woodstock: Princeton University Press.

Marcus, J. E., & Cushman, P. (1982). Ethnographies as Texts. *Annual Review of Anthropology, 11*, 25–69.

Melville, K. (1972). *Communes in the Counter Culture: Origins, Theories, Styles of Life.* New York: William Morrow and Company.

Merz-Benz, P-U. (1991). Die begriffliche Architektonik von „Gemeinschaft und Gesellschaft". In L. Clausen & C. Schlüter (Eds.), *Hundert Jahre »Gemeinschaft und Gesellschaft«. Ferdinand Tönnies in der internationalen Diskussion* (pp. 31–64). Opladen: Leske+Budrich.

Noddings, N. (1984). *Caring: A Feminine Approach to Ethics and Moral Education.* London: University of California Press.

Paterson, T. (2012). Switzerland's "Dementiaville" Designed to Mirror the Past. *Independent.co.uk.* Retrieved March 3, 2016, from http://www.independent.co.uk/news/world/europe/switzerlands-dementiaville-designed-to-mirrorthe-past-6293712.html

Pickering, M. (2009). *Auguste Comte: Volume 3: An Intellectual Biography.* Cambridge: Cambridge University Press.

Pols, J. (2012). *Care at a Distance.* Amsterdam: Amsterdam University Press.

Rosenhan, D. (1973). On Being Sane in Insane Places. *Science, 179*(4070), 250–258.

Smith, D. E. (1974). The Social Construction of Documentary Reality. *Sociological Inquiry, 44*(4), 257–268.

Tagliabue, J. (2012). Taking on Dementia with the Experiences of Normal Life. *Nytimes.com*. Retrieved March 3 2016, from http://www.nytimes.com/2012/04/25/world/europe/netherlands-hogewey-offers-normal-life-to-dementia-patients.html?_r=0

Tönebön Stiftung. (2016). Tönebön Stiftung—Ihr Partner Im Alter. *toeneboen-stiftung.de*. Retrieved March 3, 2016, from http://www.toeneboen-stiftung.de/

Tönnies, F. (2001 [1887]). *Tönnies: Community and Civil Society* (J. Harris & M. Hollis, Trans.). Cambridge: Cambridge University Press.

Townsend, P. (1952). The Purpose of the Institution. In C. Tibbits & W. Donahue (Eds.), *Social and Psychological Aspects of Aging* (pp. 378–399). New York: Columbia University Press.

Vivium Zorggroep. (2016). Verpleeghuis Hogewey. *vivium.nl*. Retrieved March 3, 2016, from www.vivium.nl/hogewey

Walther, M. (1991). Gemeinschaft und Gesellschaft bei Ferdinand Tönnies und in der Sozialphilosophie des 17. Jahrhunderts oder: Von Althusius über Hobbes zu Spinoza—und zurück. In L. Clausen & C. Schlüter (Eds.), *Hundert Jahre »Gemeinschaft und Gesellschaft«. Ferdinand Tönnies in der internationalen Diskussion* (pp. 83–106). Opladen: Leske+Budrich.

Weinberg, D. (2005). *Of Others Inside: Insanity, Addiction, and Belonging in America*. Philadelphia: Temple University Press.

Weiner, M. F., & Lipton, A. M. (2009). *The American Psychiatric Publishing Textbook of Alzheimer's Disease and Other Dementias*. Arlington: American Psychiatric Publishing.

Zola, I. K. (1972). Medicine as an Institution of Social Control. *The Sociological Review, 20*, 487–504.

Open Access This chapter is licensed under the terms of the Creative Commons Attribution 4.0 International License (http://creativecommons.org/licenses/by/4.0/), which permits use, sharing, adaptation, distribution and reproduction in any medium or format, as long as you give appropriate credit to the original author(s) and the source, provide a link to the Creative Commons license and indicate if changes were made.

The images or other third party material in this chapter are included in the chapter's Creative Commons license, unless indicated otherwise in a credit line to the material. If material is not included in the chapter's Creative Commons license and your intended use is not permitted by statutory regulation or exceeds the permitted use, you will need to obtain permission directly from the copyright holder.

Regulation as an Obstacle to Care? A Care-Ethical Evaluation of the Regulation on the Use of Seclusion Cells in Psychiatric Care in Flanders (Belgium)

Tim Opgenhaffen

Introduction

> They came. Too late. They were angry. […] I was not the only one on this unit. They cannot wait on me hand and foot. They left me there just like that. And no, I could not get a slice of bread. Breakfast is at 7:30. […] I looked upwards, to a dimmed spotlight, to the red light of the camera, and to the two sprinklers. Would they spray water in case of fire? Or gas? (Froyen 2014, p. 37)

In her diary, Brenda Froyen—who was treated for a postpartum psychosis—describes her experiences in a seclusion cell shortly after being admitted to a psychiatric hospital. She compares the practice of solitary confinement in seclusion cells with the depersonalizing techniques used in concentration camps. This is an implicit reference to Tzvetan Todorov,

T. Opgenhaffen (✉)
Institute for Social Law, Katholieke Universiteit Leuven, Leuven, Belgium

© The Author(s) 2018

F. Krause, J. Boldt (eds.), *Care in Healthcare*,
https://doi.org/10.1007/978-3-319-61291-1_9

who described the deprivation of clothing, the reduction of the victims to their animal-like basic needs, the loss of names, the large scale and the avoidance of direct communication as means to neutralize the call for help visible on the face of the other (Froyen 2014, pp. 37–39; Todorov 1999, pp. 158–177).[1]

From a care-ethical perspective, however, recognizing and responding to this call is vital. Care ethics stresses the fragile aspects of life and focuses on the interdependence and relations between the actors, thereby aiming to improve the moral integrity within these relationships (Bowden 2000, p. 39; Engster 2004, p. 114; Herring 2013, p. 14; Sander-Staudt and Hamington 2011, p. IX; Slote 2007, pp. 10–12; Tjong Tjin Tai 2007, pp. 15–26). According to Tronto, care is an ongoing process of interconnected phases. The first is to notice that care is necessary, which is to care about. Ethically, this requires attentiveness. Second, one must assume responsibility for the identified need, and thus take care of. Therefore, care requires responsibility. The third phase requires the caregiver to actually respond to the need, which means he should give care. Ethically, this calls for competence. Fourth, an observation of, and a judgement on, the response of the object of care is demanded. This is what Tronto calls care-receiving, an act for which responsiveness is needed. Recently, Tronto added a fifth phase, caring with, which requires consistency between the previous phases and the democratic commitments to justice, equality and freedom (Edwards 2009, pp. 234 f.; Tronto 1993, pp. 100–126; Tronto 2013, pp. 22–24).[2]

From this perspective, depersonalized “care” is thus no care at all. According to Froyen, the obscuring nature of institutions and regulations distracts nurses from assessing and responding to needs. Therewith, she experienced in practice what care ethicists often claim: principles and rules of action are not always the right manual for human(e) and caring behaviour (Koehn 1998, p. 26; Noddings 1984, pp. 5 f.).

This is where the legal scholar turns up. From a care perspective, his hunger for equality, universality, objectivity and positivistic rationality has a suspicious undertone.[3] Via a rephrased version of Todorov’s depersonalization thesis, this contribution tests whether the current Flemish regulation on the use of seclusion cells as a coercive measure is an obstacle for care and verifies what could be a supporting role for regulation on solitary confinement. Regulation is interpreted broadly and does not only include rules issued by the Flemish (Belgian) government ("external regulation") but also written rules issued by psychiatric hospitals ("internal regulation"). For the internal regulations, we rely on quality manuals of Flemish psychiatric hospitals and inspection reports of the Flemish Care Inspectorate (Zorginspectie 2015). When preparing this contribution, the nine inpatient psychiatric hospitals in the province of Flemish Brabant were asked to send their internal regulations on the use of seclusion cells. Five hospitals sent sufficient information. This contribution therefore does not give a comprehensive overview of all regulation(s), but points out some trends.

Depersonalizing Regulation?

In a first step, I slightly adapt and generalize the above-described characteristics of depersonalization to make it a touchstone for regulation on seclusion in inpatient psychiatric hospital care. Seclusion is defined as a type of solitary confinement whereby a patient resides in a specially designed locked room without his consent (Broeders van Liefde 1995; Steinert and Lepping 2009, p. 136; Voskes et al. 2014, p. 766). This contribution starts from the premise that seclusion might be executed in a caring way (Van Den Hooff and Goossensen 2013; Verkerk 1999; Voskes et al. 2014).[4] Care is proposed as the counterpart to depersonalization. Thereby, the definition for care in health care as set out in this volume is applied: "Care in health care is a set of relational actions that take place in an institutional context with the aim to create, maintain, improve or restore well-being".[5] Consequently, if one cares about care when using seclusion cells, this definition should be met.

Deprivation of Personal Belongings ("Deprivation of Clothing")

> I was wearing a deep blue, shapeless apron on my naked body. (Froyen 2014, p. 34)

Clothing and personal belongings are an expression of humanity. In the event of seclusion, however, patients must often hand them over for safety reasons (Kontio et al. 2012). In Flanders, Belgium, there are no external rules on patients' rights during seclusion (see Put et al. 2003), and the inspection authority rarely looks into the content of hospital procedures. Consequently, whether clothing and personal belongings have to be turned in is up to the psychiatric hospitals themselves. They internally regulate the issue in quality manuals. In the five different manuals, four provisions can be distinguished: (1) clothing and personal belongings must be handed over, (2) they must be handed over, unless there is no risk involved, (3) they need not be handed over, unless risk is involved; or (4) whether they are handed over is decided in the individual treatment plan.

The perspective of care does not object to safety rules, though it opposes the possibly categorical character of these rules, requiring unconditional obedience in every single case (Tjong Tjin Tai 2007, pp. 258–259). Categorical rules should be avoided for at least two reasons: First, they gloss over the complexity of care (Koehn 1998, p. 40; Sevenhuijsen 1998, p. 115). While in many specific situations, depriving a patient of clothing and personal belongings might be desirable or even necessary, it is imaginable that in some cases, this might have a counterproductive effect. Second, and more importantly, a categorical rule skips the role of nursing staff. The road to answering the question how to meet one's caring responsibilities in the best possible way—and thus to "care"—is closed down by categorical rules (Noddings 1984, p. 51, p. 56; Fisher 1995, p. 200). Consequently, a quality manual not drawing upon the responsibility and engagement of the caregiver is not a caring manual (Voskes et al. 2014, p. 771). For care ethics, a manual must offer guidance, but may not overrule the responsibility aspect of the patient-caregiver relationship (Edwards 2009, p. 234; Tronto 1993, p. 137).

Alienation ("Reducing the Victims to Their Animal-Like Basic Needs")

> I resisted like a threatened animal, a lioness, a beast. That's the way they have treated me.
>
> It was a dark room, a room of only a few square meters. (Froyen 2014, p. 34)

The content of regulation or a wrongful dealing with it might lead to alienation (Jeandarme 2010, p. 149); the patient is not, in the first place, perceived as a human being but, for example, as a problem. In the regulations, danger is inherently linked to seclusion (Sabbe and Bervoets 2010, p. 197). For example, in the external regulation, there is no specific rule on involuntary treatment or involuntary measures in psychiatry (Rotthier 2012, p. 295). Therefore, open norms not specifically linked to psychiatry have to be applied. These norms justify seclusion if there is a serious risk (when a patient's life or health is seriously endangered or if there is a serious risk for the integrity of third parties) (Veys 2008, pp. 132–138).[6] In Flemish external regulation, risk aversion is the only legally valid goal (Omzendbrief 1991). The reason for it is fairly straightforward and well-intended: as a consequence of the client-centred concept of autonomy underlying the Belgian patients' rights act, seclusion is one of the most far-reaching invasions on the freedom of choice, with a direct influence on a person's privacy and integrity. Therefore, seclusion must be the last resort (Veys 2008, p. 137; Omzendbrief 1991).

Care ethicists have often criticized this biomedical concept of autonomy for its wrongful overlap with an independently made decision (Cardol et al. 2002; Gilligan 1982, p. 71; Noddings 1984, pp. 359–362, 2002, pp. 109–117). Through this interpretation, care becomes a sign of dependency—opposed to autonomy (Tjong Tjin Tai 2007, p. 67; Tronto 1993, p. 140). This negative concept of autonomy overlooks the essence of personhood as defined by relationships and interdependence. For care ethics, care is not opposed to autonomy, but leads to it (Janssens et al. 2004, p. 454; Tjong Tjin Tai 2007, p. 365; Verkerk 1999, 2001). Not autonomy itself, but the capacity to attain it must be the focus (Noddings 2002, p. 110; Slote 2007, p. 62; Tjong Tjin Tai 2007, p. 68). This viewpoint on autonomy is expressed in Driessen's contribution (Chapter "Sociomaterial Will-Work. Aligning Daily Wanting in Dutch Dementia Care") in this volume, where she describes the process of socio-material will-work. As Verkerk notes, coercion that aims at restoring autonomy might be care. Non-interference does not necessarily respect a patient's autonomy (Herring 2013, p. 174; Verkerk 1999, p. 366; Voskes et al. 2014[7]). Although a care perspective would come to the same conclusion as regulation—seclusion will always go with a certain degree of danger and will be a last resort—it perceives the patient radically different. It is not in the first place about risk aversion but about restoring a person's capacity to act autonomously.

As a consequence, care as a set of relational actions—a central aspect of the *care in health care* definition—might be obscured by a regulatory discourse based on danger (Fisher 1995, p. 194; Gregory 2010, p. 2276). The patient might be reduced to, and objectified via, the danger he causes (see, e.g. Desai 2010, p. 89; Du Plessis 2013, p. 426; Fisher 1995, p. 200).[8] Internally, this is clear in most of the manuals that contain step-by-step analyses of the risk for both patients and personnel during seclusion. Although in a manual these aspects are of major importance, the care perspective is not about a patient's dangerousness, but about his well-being. The goal of risk aversion is part of this well-being, though subordinate to the goal postulated by care ethics: the restoration of the self (Koehn 1998, p. 456). Only one manual states that the prior goal is restoration, which comprises risk aversion. All other manuals as well as inspection reports merely focus on risk and may thereby result in alienation.

Reduction to Procedure ("Loss of Name")

> No, I could not get a piece of bread. Breakfast was at seven thirty. I had had nothing to eat for over 18 hours. I was hungry, I was thirsty. (Froyen 2014, p. 37)

Procedural rules might detract a caregiver's attention from the actual patient. This is an often heard statement linked to the so-called rising role of regulation in the domain of care (Put and Van Assche 2013). Although it is not substantiated that the role of regulation in Flanders has increased over the past decades (Put and Van Assche 2013), it is worth to cast a glance at the procedural burden of seclusion. The registration burden imposed by Flemish external regulation is rather low (Janssen et al. 2014[9]; Rotthier 2012, pp. 311 f.). Although hospitals must register the duration of and reason for seclusion, there is no central register (Sabbe and Bervoets 2010, p. 198; Omzendbrief 1991).[10] From a legal perspective, this implies a low level of protection: the inspection agency is not aware of individual cases, nor is there a specific complaints procedure (see Rotthier 2012, pp. 342–352, for the general complaint procedures). Internally, manuals often require a higher burden for registration, especially during seclusion. Every observation must be put down in writing, though one quality manual explicitly warns not to use subjective terms—which care-ethically is questionable (Voskes et al. 2014, p. 771).

In addition, external regulation prescribes that the role of the institution and its nursing staff is to correctly execute the decision to seclude made by the physician. In liability law, the physician might be held liable for a bad decision on seclusion, the nursing staff for a bad execution of this decision (e.g. Swennen 2003, pp. 57 f.; Van Noppen 2013/2014; Veys 2005/2006; Omzendbrief 1991).[11] This implies a fragmentation of the procedure and a division of responsibilities based on liability law. This is translated into quality manuals, in which nurses are not allowed to decide on the modalities of seclusion. Therefore, especially when a clear division of responsibilities is combined with strict manuals prescribing a caregiver's behaviour, care might be reduced to the implementation of orders, which is also demonstrated in the contribution of Pei-Yi Liu in this volume.

Despite of this fragmentation in external regulation, manuals stress that the physician consults other team members prior to making a decision. This is preferable from the viewpoint of care, as a rupture in the phases of care is potentially prevented (Tjong Tjin Tai 2007, p. 326). In this context, Tronto incites institutions to develop a rhetorical space where conflicts on the interpretation of needs might be discussed (Tronto 2010, p. 168). For her, dealing with conflicts through dialogue is essential for caring institutions.

Normalization of Seclusion ("Large Scale")

> Many psychiatric hospitals apply rules which state that patients who arrive at night automatically end up in the seclusion cell. It is some kind of a security measure due to the limited number of personnel. That is what happened to me. (Froyen 2014, p. 121)

Within a care trajectory, seclusion might seem a necessary step. The quality manual of one of the hospitals seems to suggest an automatic equation of urgency with danger, which in case of an emergency admission might lead to a low burden for seclusion. Moreover, the decision on urgency is made elsewhere and is possibly not reassessed. Overall, however, quality manuals suggest the last resort character of the measure (Omzendbrief 1991). Despite of this last resort character, seclusion seems to be applied quite frequently. Although there is no central record in Belgium, when inspection reports call a prevalence of 15% of the admitted patients relatively low, this might give an indication.[12]

Moreover, Belgium is one of the only countries in the world where seclusion in psychiatric care is at the same time combined with other coercive measures, for example, fixation (Bowers 2015). It is unclear whether and to what degree regulation has an influence on seclusion and fixation rates. Nevertheless, there is an ambiguity in Flemish external regulation. On the one hand, the technical aspects of seclusion are regulated: the presence of seclusion cells is a criterion for recognition (Rotthier 2012, p. 308),[13] possible coercive measures must be mentioned in the hospital rules,[14] registration is obligatory (Omzendbrief 1991),[15] those who are responsible are appointed (Rotthier 2012, p. 312),[16] and so on. On the other hand, it is not specifically regulated who may be secluded (Rotthier 2012, p. 295). Consequently, regulation determines that cells must be present, but not in which cases these cells could or should be used.

From a care-ethical perspective, the absence of concrete and strict rules regulating caregivers' behaviour may be applauded. Norms create a rational and objective framework, wherein care may be reduced to solving "a problem" (Noddings 1984, p. 24). There are two arguments, however, for why in this case the presence of a clear legal outlook or vision—and thus at least a minimum level of regulation specifically on seclusion—is necessary to enhance care. First, as demonstrated above, open and alienating norms based on risk dominate the decision nowadays.[17] These open norms do not only aim at problem-solving actions, they also problematize the patient himself. Open norms, without a clear perspective on the patient's well-being, might make things worse. Second, the absence of a clear perspective on seclusion, combined with the obligatory presence of seclusion cells, might lead to "defensive care" (Ankaert 2007, p. 9; Rom et al. 2006, p. 163). The psychological impact of liability law on caring practice must not be underestimated. Although care is a combination of an orientation and an action, liability law focuses on the latter (Tjong Tjin Tai 2007, p. 264). Psychiatric hospitals have a duty to protect residents from harming themselves or others. Jurisprudence accepts that a hospital can only commit itself to do everything that can be reasonably expected, but cannot be bound to the result (Veys 2005/2006).[18] Since, in case of involuntary admissions, danger is a requirement for admission, judges reasonably expect more.[19] Nursing staff—who are often unfamiliar with liability law (e.g. Scheepmans et al. 2011, p. 59)—might believe that in these cases, seclusion is what judges reasonably expect. An "if something happens" train of thought might lower the barrier to turn to seclusion (see, e.g. Van der Zwan et al. 2011, p. 125).[20]

I do not maintain that Belgian judges prefer seclusion. They do not have an *a priori* preference for it, nor do they reject it.[21] For judges, the criterion is that whatever is chosen has to be well considered. Noddings remarks that "when we care, we should, ideally, be able to present reasons for our action/inaction which would persuade a reasonable, disinterested observer that we have acted on behalf of the cared-for" (Noddings 1984, p. 23). The judge as a reasonable, disinterested observer tests whether the caregiver has acted as a good housefather. If a hospital aims to reduce coercion in a reasonable and well-considered way, judges take this into account.[22] Seclusion is, moreover, not necessarily a way to limit liability (Van Noppen 2013/2014). On the contrary, badly executed seclusion might lead to liability as well (Directoraat-generaal Basisgezondheidszorg en Crisisbeheer 2007, p. 7).[23] Defensive care is thus a wrongful argument for seclusion.

What I do assert, however, is that for mostly not-legally educated nursing staff, the presence of seclusion cells combined with a vague, danger-based legal criterion and a falsely perceived liability-sword might lead to normalization. Therefore (knowledge of) a clear regulatory outlook would enhance care.

Avoidance of Direct Communication ("Avoidance of Direct Communication")

> It was dark, except for the red flickering light of the camera. *Smile, you're on candid camera.* (Froyen 2014, p. 122)

Over the last decades, surveillance technologies have found acceptance in care, even to the extent that all quality manuals refer to the use of visual and audio surveillance technologies. Externally, the use of these technologies in seclusion cells is not regulated—one could even ask oneself whether their usage does not go against general privacy laws. For the inspection organ, their presence is neither required nor advised against. In the risk-based regulatory framework, the use of surveillance technology is justified for reasons of safety (interestingly, the issue of privacy is not even raised) (Desai 2010; Stolovy et al. 2015, p. 276). Empirical literature, however, warns of the danger related to applying surveillance technology in a discourse of risk and safety, since technology might shift the already fragile balance between care and safety in inpatient psychiatric care (Desai 2010, p. 89) and lead to a Foucaultian surveillance climate (Du Plessis 2013, p. 430; Holmes 2001). Moreover, cameras might reinforce the previously mentioned alienating effects by creating a culture of fear (Jacob and Holmes 2011, p. 110).

However, inspection reports state very clearly that these technologies cannot function as a substitute for direct communication between the patient and the caregiver. Direct observation and communication remain essential. Nonetheless, for inspection, the reason for that is, again, safety, as cameras do not register everything. Consequently, again, not the patient, but danger and safety is focused upon.

Direct communication is not necessarily ruled out by the presence of surveillance technology. All quality manuals state that caregivers should regularly—the minimum intervals are internally regulated—visit the patient. On this point, external regulation requires intensified supervision.[24] Three manuals consider visual and verbal contact to be supportive of the caregiver's surveillance task. The two other manuals see communication as a way to contribute to the well-being of the patient. One of the manuals even stresses the importance of follow-up care and a dialogue with the patient.

Towards a Supporting Role for Regulation

In the analysis above, I introduced care via a back door: when testing regulation on possibly depersonalizing effects, care—as opposed to depersonalization—automatically pops up. However—except for categorical manuals and top down internal regulation—most of the depersonalizing effects are not due to regulation itself, but due to a type of institutional care where regulation wrongfully takes the first place. In this part, I aim to reconcile care and regulation, first by pointing at how—from a care perspective—regulation might create obstacles for care and second, by elaborating on how these obstacles might be overcome.

Depersonalization Versus Care

As demonstrated, there are a number of depersonalizing aspects stemming from regulation that should worry a caregiver. With this, I do not want to assert that regulation is intentionally drafted to generate depersonalizing effects. I do not want to claim either that seclusion leads to depersonalization in the sense that caregivers necessarily act in an inhumane way. What I do maintain, however, is that (wrongfully dealing with) certain aspects of regulation might unintentionally obscure care and that this might *at least* give the patient a feeling of being depersonalized (see, e.g. Meehan et al. 2004).

The possibly depersonalizing effect of regulation stands out against the background of Tronto's phased practice of care (Tronto 1993, pp. 100–126). First, care requires noticing the need to care [Caring About]. Regulation might distract caregivers from this need. A focus on danger—the patient must be undressed, observed and guarded—implies deviating from the reason for a patient's presence in the hospital, restoring the self. Legally, the moral element of attentiveness (needs) is reduced to alertness (danger) (Bowden 1997, pp. 113–114; Jacob and Holmes 2011; Tronto 1993, pp. 134–135). Second, caregivers must assume responsibility for the needs they have noticed [Taking Care Of]. If a caregiver believes there is nothing to do about it, the patient is not taken care of. Regulation might arouse the feeling that seclusion is the only possible option, for example, because of categorical quality manuals, the distance between the caregiver and the patient or a fear for liability. Legally, the moral element of responsibility is reduced to the obligation to control the damage.

Third, the caregiver must actually respond to the need [Care-giving]. Even if a caregiver cares about and takes care of a patient, the risk of not being able to meet a patient's needs is inherent. For example, a nurse might see a patient's needs and might feel responsible for them, but in the end, he has to implement a physician's decisions or has to follow strict quality manuals (Tronto 1993, p. 109). Moral competence is then reduced to legal incompetence. Fourth, care requires an observation of, and a judgement on, the response of the object of care [Care-receiving]. As regulation might obscure the prior phases, adequate responsiveness is under pressure, since the vulnerability of the patient is looked at from the perspective of danger rather than well-being. The actual needs of the patient are obscured in the first place. Moral responsiveness is turned into legal insusceptibility.

Immanent Care, Transcendent Regulation

Despite the risk that concepts such as danger and liability might overshadow care, no single care ethicist claims we should get rid of regulation. Even Noddings states that regulation is not bad, as long as it does not oblige caregivers to prematurely switch to a "rational-objective mode" (Noddings 1984, p. 26). Recently, Tronto added the requirement that "needs and the way they are met are consistent with democratic commitments to justice, equality, and freedom for all", as a fifth phase of care [Caring With] (Tronto 1993, p. 171, 2013, p. 23). This is not only a clear message for caregivers to act in line with democratic commitments but also for democracy—and thus regulation—to be "caring". How, then, should the relationship between regulation and care be perceived in the case of seclusion?

In his doctoral thesis, I believe Tjong Tjin Tai gives a clue when he demonstrates that acting out of disposition and acting out of duty are not opposing, but alternating viewpoints at two different moments in time: duty is what comes afterwards, at the level of justification, but has no influence on the prior disposition for care itself (Tjong Tjin Tai 2007, p. 249). I maintain that the same is true for regulation: while regulation is (and should be) omnipresent in the domain of care, it should be invisible during the act of caring itself (Koehn 1998, pp. 6–7; Noddings 1984, p. 26; Robertson and Walter 2007, p. 210). Where care is immanent, regulation should be transcendent. Therewith I do not mean to say that caregivers should be unconscious of regulation: caregivers should certainly be aware of, and capable of dealing with, the regulatory framework (in advance). The act of caring itself, however, must not be subject to constant regulatory concern. This involves an appeal to both regulation and care.

An Appeal to Regulation

There should be a smooth overlap between the way care is provided and the regulation dealing with it, as implied by Tronto's caring democracy. This viewpoint has clear implications for the content and form of the regulatory framework on seclusion. Thereby, the functions of regulation serve as a stepping stone.[25]

First, regulation coordinates human behaviour [regulatory function], including in the domain of care. In the event of seclusion, this function is nowadays translated into quality manuals. Coordination, however, is not necessarily the same as determination. As demonstrated in Section "Deprivation of Personal Belongings ("Deprivation of Clothing")"and Section "Avoidance of Direct Communication ("Avoidance of Direct Communication")", manuals can be drafted in a categorical way—passing over the caring disposition and thus turning care into a problem-solving action—or in an open way, pointing at what should minimally be done, but leaving room for more (Noddings 1984, p. 55; Voskes et al. 2014). For good care, these quality manuals are nothing more than helpful guidelines—good practices—that do not stand in the way of a caring disposition and that in exceptional circumstances could be set aside or at least be discussed (see Section "Reduction to Procedure ("Loss of Name")") (Tjong Tjin Tai 2007, p. 259; Voskes et al. 2014).

Second, regulation provides for legal guarantees and legal protection [protective function]. For the moment, external regulation offers little or no protection to secluded patients: the legal position of psychiatric patients is not regulated. Even though they may draw certain rights from general norms—for example, general privacy rights—it is difficult to challenge a seclusion. Consequently, from a regulative perspective, seclusion is not over-, but rather under-regulated. A care perspective would not oppose more protective regulation, as long as this does not lead to an excessive procedural burden. In fact, care as a practice stemming from a caring disposition should not even notice the existence of a protection system. As long as there is a caring disposition and care is provided according to the five phases, the protective function of regulation stays in the background. Once care as a relational and dialogical type of protection goes awry, regulatory protection is brought into the open (Koehn 1998, p. 40).

Third, regulation resolves conflicts [dispute solving function]. Under Section "Normalization of Seclusion ("Large Scale")", we have already demonstrated that a sole focus on this function might lead to distortions and even more seclusion. Nevertheless, in parallel with the protective function, conflict resolution should be invisible and superfluous for care. Within (the five phases of) care, disputes are dealt with dialogically and outside of the regulatory framework. Tronto's rhetorical space in institutional care is a textbook example (Tronto 2010, p. 168). Besides, the shift towards alternative dispute resolution in law might contribute to the preservation and restoration of a caring relationship (Sevenhuijsen 1998, p. 116; Tronto 2010, pp. 166–169). Only when there is a rupture in care itself and care is, as a consequence, out of reach, classical regulatory dispute resolution turns up (Koehn 1998, p. 40, pp. 51–52).

Fourth, regulation expresses cultural meaning and societal values [symbolic function] and consequently enters into Tronto's caring democracy, where justice is reframed as *caring with* for the common good (Tronto 2013, p. 182). The protective values currently underlying the regulation on seclusion—autonomy, integrity and safety—should be subordinate to and assessed from the perspective of care as a central value in a democracy or a democratic institution (Koehn 1998, pp. 34–35; Sevenhuijsen 1998, p. 110–113; Slote 2007, pp. 94–96; Tronto 2013, p. 159, p. 164). The current rupture between danger and autonomy obscures the perspective of care (see Section "Normalization of Seclusion ("Large Scale")").[26] It would be better to explicitly regulate seclusion, whereby its role as a protective measure should be exceeded and turned into the goal of restoring the self in a context of interdependency. Legally, this implies that seclusion should be categorized and regulated as "forced treatment", rather than as a "safety measure". This requires a turnover of the concept of autonomy.

An Appeal to Care

On the side of care, caregivers should not be overwhelmed or blinded by regulation. Many potentially depersonalizing consequences of regulation—the concepts of danger and protection, the fragmentation of responsibility, the level of abstraction, the stress on actions rather than dispositions and so on—cannot be shove aside. These aspects may, however, not paralyse care. Depersonalization is not a feature of regulation, but a feature of an institutional care setting where regulation wrongfully takes the first place. Although not all aspects of regulation are supportive of care, even in its present form, regulation is mostly not opposite to care. On the contrary, some quality manuals even support and fuel a care-ethical reflection. Moreover, regulation might have a supportive function for care, for example, via the creation of a forum for interpersonal dialogue or via a turnover of the safety perception in psychiatric care (De Benedictis et al. 2011).

Conclusion

Through the concept of depersonalization, this contribution has demonstrated that regulation might be an obstacle to care for secluded patients. Especially when rules are categorical or have a vague outlook, are fragmentizing or aimed at problems rather than persons, care might be endangered. However, we should not abolish all regulation or perceive it all sceptically. Nor should we turn care ethics into rules, since the disposition for care can, essentially, not be regulated.

This contribution maintains that, in the domain of seclusion, regulation and care can fruitfully co-exist if, on the regulatory side, the functions of the regulation are tailored to the needs of care and, on the side of care, regulation is not wrongfully perceived as *the* benchmark. For seclusion in Flanders, Belgium, this requires a mental shift in attitudes towards care. Regulation is not at the centre, but at the outskirts of care. At these edges, regulation aims to (1) support—not obstruct—care via references to good practices. There, the role of an open, dialogical and well-thought-out internal regulation is essential. Furthermore, regulation aims to (2) intervene when care goes awry. Even today, in most cases, care should not worry about regulation: the legal requirement of risk aversion, for example, does not contradict the caring requirement to restore the self.

The possibly depersonalizing effects of regulation on seclusion are unfolded in the way care and regulation deal with one another, not in regulation as such. Nonetheless, rethinking regulation, especially at the external level, would be supportive to care. In a regulatory framework that cares about care, seclusion should be turned into a well-regulated type of forced treatment—rather than a protective measure—with an outlook towards more autonomy and a clear—though not overburdening—protective framework, by which conflicts can be resolved when things go awry. This type of regulation would not be an obstacle but an added value for care.

Notes

1. Quotes from the work of Froyen are Translated by the author. Froyen referred to Todorov indirectly via the categorization made in Pollefeyt (1997, p. 99–101).
2. For a similar application to seclusion, see Voskes et al. (2014, p. 771).
3. See, for example, A-M. Mol, "The logic of care", presentation at the workshop Caring about Care, Amsterdam, University of Amsterdam, 8 Feb. 2016.
4. *Contra* Driessen (Chapter "Sociomaterial Will-Work. Aligning Daily Wanting in Dutch Dementia Care"), in this volume.
5. Cf. chapter *Introduction* (Chapter "Understanding Care. Introductory Remarks") of this volume.
6. Combination of Art. 8, §5 and Art. 15, §2 Patients' rights law, Art. 416 and Art. 422*bis* Penal Law Code and legal necessity in legal doctrine and jurisprudence.
7. On how the five minutes before seclusion may defuse the situation.
8. See, for example, *Vragen en Antwoorden Vlaams Parlement* 1995–1996, 7 May 1996, 13 (vr. 47 J. Stassen).

9. The registration burden is low, especially when compared to, for example, the Netherlands.
10. See Art. 5, §2 Royal Order 8 July 1991 ter uitvoering van artikel 36 van de wet van 26 juni 1990 betreffende de bescherming van de persoon van de geesteszieke, *BS* 26 juli 1991. Further referred to as RO 8 July 1991.
11. For case law, see Rb. Tongeren 15 May 1995, *Rechtskundig Weekblad* (1996–97) 362; Kh. Brussels 31 May 2005, Tijdschrift voor Gezondheidsrecht 5 (2005–06) 39.
12. Compare to 11% in the Netherlands (Steinert et al. 2010) and a rise to almost 20% in case of psychosis (Janssen et al. 2014, p. 133).
13. Art. 5, §1 RO 8 July 1991.
14. Art. 3 RO 8 July 1991.
15. Art. 5, §2 RO 8 July 1991.
16. Attachement 1 of the Royal Order of 18 June 1990 houdende vaststelling van de lijst van de technische verpleegkundige verstrekkingen en de lijst van de handelingen die door een arts aan beoefenaars van de verpleegkunde kunnen worden toevertrouwd, alsmede de wijze van uitvoering van die verstrekkingen en handelingen en de kwalificatievereisten waaraan de beoefenaars van de verpleegkunde moeten voldoen, *BS* 27 July 1990.
17. Combination of Art. 8, §5 and Art. 15, §2 Patients' rights law, Art. 416 and Art. 422*bis* Penal Law Code and legal necessity in legal doctrine and jurisprudence.
18. For case law, see Ghent 10 March 2011, *Tijdschrift voor Gezondheidsrecht* 3 (2013–14)189; *contra* Rb. Tongeren 15 September 2004, *Limb. Rechtsl.* 2004, 283.
19. See case law: Antwerp 11 October 2005, *Limburgs Rechtsleven* 3 (2006) 179.
20. Also see Haeusermann (Chapter "The Dementia Village—Between Community and Society") in this volume.
21. For case law, see Vred. Eeklo 12 January 1995, *Tijdschrift voor Gentse rechtspraak* (1995) 171–172; Antwerp 19 January 1998, *Tijdschrift voor Gezondheidsrecht* (1998–99) 312; See parallel for fixation Corr. Bruges 2 May 2005, *Tijdschrift voor Gezondheidsrecht* 3 (2007–08) 228 and case-law note Veys (2007–08), pp. 224–225.
22. For case law, see Antwerp 6 November 2003, *Tijdschrift voor Gezondheidsrecht* (2003–04) 40; Antwerp 11 October 2005, *Limburgs Rechtsleven* 3 (2006) 179.
23. For example in case law on fixation: Ghent 10 September 1997, *Tijdschrift voor Gezondheidsrecht* (1999–00) 130–131.

24. Art. 5, §2 RO 8 July 1991.
25. The four functions of regulation are derived from Claes et al. 2009, pp. 5–11.
26. See a similar debate in the Netherlands in, for example, Arends and Frederiks 2006.

References

Ankaert, E. (2007). Jeugdzorg in de ban van schuldig hulpverzuim. *Tijdschrift voor Sociale Interventie, 16*(3), 5–12.

Arends, L. A. P., & Frederiks, B. J. M. (2006). Vrijheidsbeperking in de psychogeriatrie en verstandelijk gehandicaptenzorg: de contouren van een nieuwe regeling. *Tijdschrift voor Gezondheidsrecht, 30*(2), 81–89.

Bowden, P. (1997). *Caring. Gender-Sensitive Ethics*. London: Routledge.

Bowden, P. (2000). An 'Ethic of Care' in Clinical Settings: Encompassing 'Feminine' and 'Feminist' Perspectives. *Nursing Philosophy, 1*(1), 36–49.

Bowers, L. (2015, December 11). *New Prospects for Peace on the Wards*. Dwang in de Psychiatrie (Oral Presentation). Brussels: Superior Health Council.

Broeders van Liefde. (1995). Afzonderen niet afzonderen. Een ethische benadering van het afzonderen van psychiatrische patiënten. *broedersvanliefde.be*. Retrieved January 9, 2017, from http://www.broedersvanliefde.be/document/ethiek/Ethisch%20advies%20GGZ%20-%20Afzonderen.pdf

Cardol, M., De Jong, B. A., & Ward, C. D. (2002). On Autonomy and Participation in Rehabilitation. *Disability and Rehabilitation, 24*(18), 970–974.

Claes, E., Devroe, W., & Keirsbilck, B. (2009). The Limits of the Law. In E. Claes, W. Devroe, & B. Keirsbilck (Eds.), *Facing the Limits of the Law* (pp. 5–11). Berlin: Springer.

De Benedictis, L., Dumais, A., Sieu, N., Mailhot, M., Létourneau, G., Tran, M. M., Stikarovska, I., Bilodeau, M., Brunelle, S., Côté, G., & Lesage, A. D. (2011). Staff Perceptions and Organizational Factors as Predictors of Seclusion and Restraint on Psychiatric Wards. *Psychiatric Services, 62*(5), 484–491.

Desai, S. (2010). Violence and Surveillance. Some Unintended Consequences of CCTV Monitoring Within Mental Health Hospital Wards. *Surveillance & Society, 8*(1), 85–92.

Directoraat-generaal Basisgezondheidszorg & Crisisbeheer. (2007). *Eindverslag technische commissie voor verpleegkunde. Werkgroep Fixatie en Isolatie*. Retrieved

January 9, 2017, from http://www.valpreventie.be/Portals/Valpreventie/Documenten/WZC/EVV_WZC_Fixatie_Techncomm.pdf

Du Plessis, R. (2013). Constructing Patient–Psychiatrist Relations in Psychiatric Hospitals. The Role of Space and Personal Action. *Social Semiotics, 23*(3), 424–443.

Edwards, S. D. (2009). Three Versions of an Ethics of Care. *Nursing Philosophy, 10*(4), 231–240.

Engster, D. (2004). Care Ethics and Natural Law Theory. Toward and Institutional Political Theory of Caring. *The Journal of Politics, 66*(1), 113–135.

Fisher, A. (1995). The Ethical Problems Encountered in Psychiatric Nursing Practice with Dangerous Mentally Ill Persons. *Scholarly Inquiry for Nursing Practice, 9*(2), 193–208.

Froyen, B. (2014). *Kortsluiting in mijn hoofd*. Antwerpen: Manteau.

Gilligan, C. (1982). *In a Different Voice*. Cambridge: Harvard University Press.

Gregory, M. (2010). Reflection and Resistance. Probation Practice and the Ethic of Care. *British Journal of Social Work, 40*(7), 2274–2290.

Herring, J. (2013). *Caring and the Law*. London: Hart Publishing.

Holmes, D. (2001). From Iron Gaze to Nursing Care. Mental Health Nursing in the Era of Panopticism. *Journal of Psychiatric and Mental Health Nursing, 8*(1), 7–15.

Jacob, J. D., & Holmes, D. (2011). The Culture of Fear. Expanding the Concept of Risk in Forensic Psychiatric Nursing. *International Journal of Culture and Mental Health, 4*(2), 106–115.

Janssen, W., Noorthoorn, E., Van de Sande, R., Nijmana, H., Smit, A., Hoogendoorn, A., Mulder, N., Voskes, Y., & Widdershoven, G. (2014). *Zes jaar Argus. Vrijheidsbeperkende interventies in de GGz in 2012 en ontwikkelingen ten opzichte van voorgaande jaren*. Retrieved January 9, 2017, from http://www.ggznederland.nl/uploads/assets/Rapport%20-%20zes%20jaar%20argus%2017062014.pdf.pdf

Janssens, M. J. P. A., Kortmann, F. A. M., Ten Have, H. A. M. J., Van Rooij, M. F. A. M., & Van Wijmen, F. C. B. (2004). Pressure and Coercion in the Care for the Addicted. Ethical Perspectives. *Journal of Medical Ethics, 30*, 453–458.

Jeandarme, I. (2010). Risicotaxaties bij psychiatrische patiënten. Risky Business. In W. Canton, L. Claes, L. Gijs, I. Jeandarme, E. Klein-Haneveld, & D. van Beek (Eds.), *De bescherming van de persoon van de geesteszieke* (pp. 143–160). Brugge: Die Keure.

Koehn, D. (1998). *Rethinking Feminist Ethics. Care, Trust and Empathy*. London: Routledge.

Kontio, R., Joffe, G., Putkonen, H., Kuosmanen, L., Hane, K., Holi, M., & Välimäki, M. (2012). Seclusion and Restraint in Psychiatry: Patients' Experiences and Practical Suggestions on How to Improve Practices and Use Alternatives. *Perspectives in Psychiatric Care, 48*(1), 16–24.

Lock, M. (1993). *Encounters with Aging: Mythologies of Menopause in Japan and North America*. London: University of California Press.

Meehan, T., Bergen, H., & Fjeldsoe, K. (2004). Staff and Patient Perceptions of Seclusion: Has Anything Changed? *Journal of Advanced Nursing, 47*(1), 33–38.

Noddings, N. (1984). *Caring: A Feminine Approach to Ethics and Moral Education*. Berkeley: University of California Press.

Noddings, N. (2002). *Starting at Home. Caring and Social Policy*. Berkeley: University of California Press.

Omzendbrief. (1991, September 23). Omzendbrief aan de Psychiatrische Ziekenhuizen en aan de Algemene Ziekenhuizen met een Psychiatrische Afdeling.

Pollefeyt, D. (1997). Auschwitz or How Good People Can Do Evil. An Ethical Interpretation of the Perpetrators and the Victims of the Holocaust in Light of the French Thinker Tzvetan Todorov. In G. J. Colijn & M. L. Littell (Eds.), *Confronting the Holocaust: A Mandate for the 21st Century?* (pp. 99–101). New York: University Press of America.

Put, J., & Van Assche, L. (2013). *Juridisering van de zorgsector. Een verkennende begrips- en fenomeenstudie*. Steunpunt Welzijn, Volksgezondheid en Gezin Rapport 11. Leuven. Retrieved January 9, 2017, from https://steunpuntwvg.be/images/rapporten-en-werknotas/juridisering-van-de-zorgsector.-een-verkennende-begrips-en-fenomeenstudie

Put, J., Verdeyen, V., & Loosveldt, G. (2003). *Gebruikersrechten in de welzijnszorg*. Brugge: Die Keure.

Robertson, M., & Walter, G. (2007). Overview of Psychiatric Ethics II: Virtue Ethics and the Ethics of Care. *Australian Psychiatry, 15*(3), 207–211.

Rom, M., Ankaert, E., & Put, J. (2006). *Over risico's en beperkingen. Juridisch onderzoek naar de positie van de consulenten van de sociale diensten van de Bijzondere Jeugdbijstand, met focus op 'aansprakelijkheid' en 'schuldig verzuim'*. Leuven: Instituut voor Sociaal Recht KU Leuven.

Rotthier, K. (2012). *Gedwongen opname van de geesteszieke. Handleiding bij de Wet Persoon Geesteszieke*. Brugge: Die Keure.

Sabbe, B., & Bervoets, C. (2010). Vrijheidsbeperking door afzondering. Een gemiste kans voor onderzoek? In B. Sabbe & C. Bervoets (Eds.), *De bescherming van de persoon van de geesteszieke* (pp. 197–207). Brugge: Die Keure.

Sander-Staudt, M., & Hamington, M. (2011). Introduction: Care Ethics and Business Ethics. In M. Sander-Staudt & M. Hamington (Eds.), *Applying Care Ethics to Business* (p. IX). Dordrecht: Springer.

Scheepmans, K., Dierckx de Casterlé, B., Paquay, L., Van Gansbeke, H., & Milisen, K. (2011). *De ervaringen van thuisverpleegkundigen bij het toepassen van vrijheidsbeperkende maatregelen. Een kwalitatieve studie*. Brussels. Retrieved January 9, 2017, from https://lirias.kuleuven.be/bitstream/123456789/425593/1/Onderzoeksrapport+VBM+K

Sevenhuijsen, S. (1998). *Citizenship and the Ethics of Care: Feminist Considerations on Justice, Morality and Politics*. London: Routledge.

Slote, M. (2007). *The Ethics of Care and Empathy*. London: Routledge.

Steinert, T., & Lepping, P. (2009). Legal Provisions and Practice in the Management of Violent Patients. A Case Vignette Study in 16 European Countries. *European Psychiatry, 24*(2), 135–141.

Steinert, T., Lepping, P., Bernhardsgrütter, R., Conca, A., Hatling, T., Janssen, W., Keski-Valkama, A., Mayoral, F., & Whittington, R. (2010). Incidence of Seclusion and Restraint in Psychiatric Hospitals. A Literature Review and Survey of International Trends. *Social Psychiatry and Psychiatric Epidemiology, 45*(9), 889–997.

Stolovy, T., Melamed, Y., & Afek, A. (2015). Video Surveillance in Mental Health Facilities. Is It Ethical? *The Israel Medical Association Journal, 17*(5), 274–276.

Swennen, F. (2003). Aansprakelijkheid van en voor geestesgestoorden. In F. Swennen (Ed.), *Bijzondere overeenkomsten. Artikelsgewijze commentaar met overzicht van rechtspraak en rechtsleer, IV. Commentaar Verbintenissenrecht, Titel III, Hfdst. 6* (pp. 57–58). Mechelen: Kluwer.

Tjong Tjin Tai, T. F. E. (2007). *Zorgplichten en zorgethiek*. Amsterdam: University of Amsterdam.

Todorov, T. (1999). *Facing the Extreme. Moral Life in the Concentration Camps*. London: Weidenfeld.

Tronto, J. (1993). *Moral Boundaries. A Political Argument for an Ethics of Care*. New York: Routledge.

Tronto, J. (2010). Creating Caring Institutions. Politics, Plurality and Purpose. *Ethics and Social Welfare, 4*(2), 158–171.

Tronto, J. (2013). *Caring Democracy. Markets, Equality, and Justice*. New York: New York University Press.

Van den Hooff, S., & Goossensen, A. (2013). How to Increase the Quality of Care During Coercive Admission? A Review of Literature. *Scandinavian Journal of Caring Science, 28*(3), 425–434.

Van der Zwan, R., Davies, L., Andrews, D., & Brooks, A. (2011). Aggression and Violence in the ED. Issues Associated with the Implementation of Restraint and Seclusion. *Health Promotion Journal of Australia, 22*(2), 124–127.

Van Noppen, W. (2013/2014). De toezichtsplicht van verzorgingsinstellingen en zorgverstrekkers bij geesteszieke patiënten met zelfmoordneigingen. *Tijdschrift voor Gezondheidsrecht, 3*, 193–195.

Verkerk, M. (1999). A Care Perspective on Coercion and Autonomy. *Bioethics, 13*(3–4), 358–368.

Verkerk, M. (2001). The Care Perspective and Autonomy. *Medicine, Health Care and Philosophy, 4*, 289–294.

Veys, M. N. (2005/2006). What's in a Name? Is de toezichtsplicht van een psychiatrische instelling op een geesteszieke een inspannings- of een resultaatsverbintenis? *Tijdschrift voor Gezondheidsrecht, 5*, 400–408.

Veys, M. N. (2007/2008). Fixatie bij bejaarden: een situering in het gezondheids- en aansprakelijkheidsrecht. *Tijdschrift voor Gezondheidsrecht, 3*, 214–227.

Veys, M. N. (2008). *Patientenrechten in de psychiatrie*. Brussels: Larcier.

Voskes, Y., Kemper, M., Landeweer, E. G. M., & Widdershoven, G. A. M. (2014). Preventing Seclusion in Psychiatry. A Care Ethics Perspective on the First Five Minutes at Admission. *Nursing Ethics, 21*, 766–773.

Zorginspectie. (2015). *Flemish Care Inspectorate*. www4wvg.vlaanderen.be. Retrieved January 9, 2017, from http://www4wvg.vlaanderen.be/wvg/zorginspectie/pages/En.aspx

Open Access This chapter is licensed under the terms of the Creative Commons Attribution 4.0 International License (http://creativecommons.org/licenses/by/4.0/), which permits use, sharing, adaptation, distribution and reproduction in any medium or format, as long as you give appropriate credit to the original author(s) and the source, provide a link to the Creative Commons license and indicate if changes were made.

The images or other third party material in this chapter are included in the chapter's Creative Commons license, unless indicated otherwise in a credit line to the material. If material is not included in the chapter's Creative Commons license and your intended use is not permitted by statutory regulation or exceeds the permitted use, you will need to obtain permission directly from the copyright holder.

Witnessing as an Embodied Practice in German Midwifery Care

Annekatrin Skeide

Introduction: Witnessing in Midwifery Care

The first birth I saw was a homebirth. At the time I was interested in becoming a midwife and I accompanied two midwives in order to get an idea of their work. They were living in my neighbouring village in the south of France and had been attending homebirths for over twenty years. It was a dark and silent night. When I arrived, the mother-to-be—I will call her Lisa—lay on her bed in white sheets. The midwife Hélène sat cross-legged at the front-side of the bed. She appeared to be relaxed and highly concentrated at the same time. Hélène smiled slightly when I arrived, but barely took her eyes off Lisa. Lisa did not seem to notice me at all. She was lying on her side breathing heavily. I remember her wearing a white t-shirt. Her body seemed to dissolve in the white sheets, while her naked arms and legs seemed to function apart from her. Every time she had a contraction, she clutched the metallic bedframe with her strong, muscular hands and the whole bed was shaken by the

A. Skeide (✉)
Human and Health Sciences, University of Bremen, Bremen, Germany

© The Author(s) 2018

F. Krause, J. Boldt (eds.), *Care in Healthcare*,
https://doi.org/10.1007/978-3-319-61291-1_10

enormous tension of her muscles. She seemed to be in great pain: at the height of a contraction she screamed deeply and desperately. Meanwhile, Hélène remained silent and immovable. Her calm comforted and irritated me at the same time. How could she leave Lisa suffering without doing anything beneath murmuring now and then that Lisa was doing very well? It seemed to be endless and circular: silence, a throaty groaning swelling to a scream accompanied by metallic rattling and silence again. Then all of a sudden the midwife moved forward to take a look between Lisa's legs. She stayed next to Lisa, telling her to breathe shortly. Holding my breath, I noticed the baby's head appearing slowly. His slick and bluish body followed easily. Lisa took her child and lay down—she seemed exhausted but suddenly very present and relieved. I was overwhelmed: still shocked by the force of Lisa's contractions which had seemed to be torturous but amazed by this unbelievable miracle I just had been part of.

Hélène was witnessing Lisa's birth: Highly attentive, she was sitting an arm's length away from Lisa who was absorbed by the enormous effort and pain of giving birth to her child. Hélène knew that everything went fine. Lisa found her own strategies of handling the birthing pain and by doing so she enacted Hélène as a witness.

In the situation described, witnessing compromises embodied[1] interrelatedness in a particular environment. The witnesses presence has to be characterized as an intervention: an activity which shapes and constitutes what happens but which is shaped and constituted by what is happening as well.

In order to elucidate why and how I use witnessing as a concept I am going to introduce juridical, religious and philosophical reflections on witnessing and connect them to midwifery practices.

In a second step, I will elaborate on witnessing in midwifery care with the help of my empirical findings. Firstly, I am going to introduce and confound two widespread stereotypes in midwifery care: the knitting midwife and the head-led woman in labour. In doing so I would like to demonstrate that witnessing signifies 'being-with' and relates to mutual obligations; I also point out the limits of witnessing. Secondly, I develop the interpretative aspect of witnessing and displaying possible consequences. Thirdly, eye-witnessing will be revealed as a practice and a state. Fourthly, I am going to introduce touch as another sensual mode of witnessing in midwifery care. Fifthly, I define and illustrate trustful witnessing. Finally, I explain how CTGs perform technological testifying. I shall reveal the limits of witnessing throughout the text. I am going to present these aspects separately for analytical purposes. Nevertheless, it hopefully becomes evident that these witnessing states and techniques are intertwined.

Juridical, Religious, Philosophical and Sociological Facets of Witnessing Applied to Midwifery Care

At first view, witnessing seems to be inseparable from the legal sphere: The witness is the third person (Lat. terstis = the third) who assisted (Derrida 2005, p. 23). A witness is called to court in order to testify. In the legal context, the witness seems to be indispensable, because he or she is supposed to be the one who actually participated in the situation he or she is expected to bear witness about without being involved. He or she is the one who knows (old Engl. witnes = knowledge, understanding) without being the one who did it. In the quest to find just judgement, clear evidence furnished by a neutral and objective observer is required. But it is also obvious that the witness cannot tell the truth because he or she is not independent, but influenced (and even transformed) by what happened, by his or her feelings and also by those assigning him or her the role of being a witness and testifying (Krämer 2011, pp. 122–125; Schmidt 2011, pp. 48 f.). Witnesses can but re-interpret situations they are involved in and so they have to be trusted. Witnessing constitutes sense and orientation (Krämer 2011, p. 128; Schmidt 2011, pp. 47–66). For being trusted the witness has to be self-conscious and responsible. Eye-witnessing is meant to furnish strong evidence not only in juridical but also in historic or religious contexts. The sense of sight is also of particular importance in certain philosophical traditions (Onfray 1992, pp. 34 f.). In rationalism, language is a fundamental medium of reason. However, Jewish and

Christian martyrs (Grk. martys = witness) testify divine truth not only through words but also through action which has to be seen (Drews and Schlie 2011, pp. 7–21).

The multidisciplinary approach to witnessing shows its epistemological ambiguity: a witness is supposed to be the third, the neutral, the observing. But being the third does not mean not being involved and related. Being neutral does not mean not feeling or not experiencing or not reflecting and not acting. Being the observer does not mean only being made up of an eyed brain.[2] Because it is situated and embodied witnessing involves trust.

The integrative active part of participating cannot be separated from the seeing and observing presence in midwifery care. Even if the midwife seems to do nothing else than observing, she actually is intervening and interpreting. As witnessing is inter-relational, the midwife is enacted as a witness too. Eye-witnessing in midwifery care has a distant and alienating potential, because it might stem from or lead to women's bodily exposure. Women feel a separation with regard to their body then. Midwives witness and testify[3] birth which can be perceived and influenced by midwives but 'happens to' childbearing women and regarding which midwives have a certain professional knowledge and experience which the childbearing woman generally does not have. The childbearing woman for her part disposes of (medical, social, corporeal etc.) knowledge and experience, too. The witnessing role is socially and politically assigned to the midwife.[4] This assignment is constantly renewed in interaction with women and families but also with colleagues, surroundings, and things. It is performative: Witnessing is established and maintained in and by acting. Legally speaking, midwives testify by doing paper work and documenting what they saw and did.

Trust is conditional in the relationship between midwives and women. The midwife is usually met as a trustworthy person in regard to her competences, her confidentiality and her good intentions. Trust is not only anticipated by mothers-to-be but also established or reinforced in reaction to the required intimate exposure of themselves, especially during birth.

Midwives are using technical aids such as the cardiotocograph (CTG) in order to produce testimonials. Technological testimonies function as providers of the objective and neutral evidence, the higher truth that the witness fails to provide. The CTG is enacted as the ideal witness, as a producer of a category of knowledge which is not partial and subjective, embedded in embodied presence, but which is total, neutral and objective. The ambiguity of witnessing becomes quite obvious when midwives use the CTG as a competitor, a colleague or a superior.

Empirical Findings

I conducted one year of ethnographical fieldwork in two midwife-led birthplaces, one obstetrical ward in a mid-sized hospital and in numerous families' homes in Northern and Eastern Germany.[5] As I introduced myself as a midwife I was quite frequently asked for my opinion about how to proceed in certain situations by the midwives[6] and often included in conversations between midwives and women.[7] Sometimes I could lend a hand, too. Usually, I made quick notes during the rare pauses, which I elaborated after having left the field site. Furthermore, I conducted about twenty guided interviews with women and midwives. I conducted fieldwork and data analysis parallel using theoretical sampling and conceptualized the data by coding and memo writing as proposed by grounded theorists (Glaser and Strauss 1971; Strauss 1987).

Witnessing as a Contractual Being-With

The role the midwife played during Lisa's birth actually illustrates the topos of the knitting midwife[8] which seems to do nothing apart from sitting and knitting. Actually, this is not the case. The knitting midwife is the sage-femme.[9] She does little *because* she knows a lot. She knits to occupy her skilful hands. Nevertheless, she sees, hears, feels and speaks. She could interrupt the knitting at any time in order to intervene actively if it would become necessary. Deciding if and when this necessity appears is crucial. The knitting midwife is "active-passive". Hélène attended Lisa's birth at Lisa's home. The domestic setting relieves midwives from pressures initiated by institutional settings such as attending several women at once, working in shifts, following clinical guidelines, being subordinated to doctors and therefore being obligated to report and follow instructions. Being a guest, Hélène depends on Lisa's permission and guidance when moving around or using anything. Lisa is all by herself, not tasking the midwife to intervene, to validate or interpret her bodily functions. Hélène's knitting midwife's role is situated in a specific configuration, which yields the knitting midwife.

Midwife Anna describes a stereotype which I have been socialized with when becoming a midwife and which I met again frequently during my fieldwork: the head-led woman in labour. The head-led woman is not able to "let her body guide her" as midwives advise. In consequence, her birth has to be medically assisted. I would like to show that these situations rather lie on relational aspects: The configuration of midwife and woman in labour has contractual implications.

Anna, a young self-employed midwife, told me about Katharina, who, as Anna told me, had been quite exhausting to attend to during her homebirth. Katharina had the impression that Anna called her "every five minutes" during the night, even though she had only had light contractions. When Anna finally got there she had been quite annoyed because Katharina "had only been at two centimetres".[10] Katharina stared at Anna continuously and expectantly. Anna said that Katharina "had not been in possession of herself [nicht bei sich war]". Instead Katharina had figuratively tried to "crawl into [hineinkriechen]" Anna. Anna felt like Katharina "wanted to get it done" by her, the midwife. Katharina for her part needed even more than the midwife's interpretative support. She appealed to her midwife to manage the pain at her place and share it with her corporeally, what Anna described as "crawl into me". In this situation, witnessing had not been possible anymore.

Apparently expectations and appeals towards the midwife's participation differ in dependence on the woman's experience of her body-in-labour (Akrich and Pasveer 2004, p. 65).[11] Katharina had been overwhelmed by her labours. She desperately appealed to the midwife to define what was happening to her in order to make it understandable and even to handle her body-in-labour in her place. The alienation

Katharina feels towards her body-in-labour cannot be mitigated by midwife Anna, because Anna is neither able to remove it nor to handle it in her place.

Midwife and childbearing woman are situated in a kind of contract: The woman in labour cannot escape from her body. She has to fulfil her role and assume the birthing process in order to allow the midwife to fulfil her professional role for her part.

In what follows, I would like to show that corporeal insecurity women perceive during pregnancy and birth can also be reassured by midwives. If midwives concede a scope of action to women and if women are actually able to make use of it, they might handle what they perceive as their dys-appearing body (Leder 1990).

Witnessing as a Reassuring Being-With

Most women undergo a feeling of uncertainty during pregnancy, birth and the postpartum stage, even if it is not the first time they are experiencing it. One main aim of the attendance by a midwife is to reassure the woman by "normalizing" her experiences. The feminine body is subject to significant changes. The usually absent body can become a *dys-appearing* body: it manifests itself as a difficult or disharmonious body. A problematic interpretation could be that life phases in which this usually happens are identified as being dysfunctional or alienating themselves (Leder 1990).

Eli had an appointment with the midwife in the early morning. She arrived crimson red and snorting, obviously suffering from her enormously big womb. The expected delivery date had been three days ago. "I'm in such a bad mood". Eli sat down straddle-legged, face-to-face to the midwife who looked at her attentively. Eli had given several false alarms because she had thought the baby would come. "I can't sleep, I have cramps and my back hurts. I have been ill for nine months. It has to come now". The midwife says that she understands her and then asks when Eli wants her child to come. "Tomorrow". she answers. "What time?" "In the morning". This would be doable with her schedule, too, the midwife says and Eli leaves apparently relieved.

The midwife acknowledges Eli's pain and legitimizes her anger by not refuting it or trying to calm her. Instead she establishes a scope of action or at least a scope of decision: Eli who had suffered from her dys-appearing body throughout the whole pregnancy is now taking the decision to give birth to her child.

Similarly, Melanie asks her midwife if it would be normal that she was having headaches very frequently since she became pregnant. Instead of answering her question the midwife asks her what helped her when she had these headaches. "Lemon oil". she answers. "Well, it's great that you found something which helps you". Actually, Melanie had already adopted a strategy to get along with her headaches. Nevertheless, she felt insecure and needed support. The midwife normalized Melanie's discomfort by evaluating her strategy.

Frequently, midwives attribute a scope of action to women during birth by encouraging them: "You're doing well!"; "Yes, keep pushing. Your feeling is completely right". Or by helping them to understand and interpret their body-in-labour and their emotional state: "You're feeling tired, huh? You would like to go home, huh? That's normal at this point. Your cervix is surely fully dilated now". External interpretation does not necessarily create alienation, but joins or integrates corporeal dys-appearances. In order to make this work women have to cooperate with their dys-appearing body and to use their scope of action.

Eye-Witnessing as an Alienating Being-With

I have described witnessing as an inter-relational practice which is situated in specific midwife-woman-body-setting-thing-time configurations. Witnessing is being-with, an active passiveness, an intervention which is associated with acknowledging a scope of action to women during pregnancy and birth. Witnessing is associated with fulfilling certain role obligations. In what follows, I would like to show a different configuration in a clinical setting in which witnessing was experienced as alienating.

Samia, who had had a lengthy birth in hospital, had been attended by several midwives and she went through all the shifts she explained. Samia told me, she felt "unsheathed [blankgezogen]" during birth and that she "really had to do circus there". In the end, this would have been "the only way to make it work". Samia had handed over responsibility: She said her head had been turned off. She simply did what she had been told knowing she was in good hands. "And at the end comes the child". Samia had neither decided who had taken care of her during her birth nor what should have been done. She describes her birth experience through a distanced perspective, qualifying herself as being at the mercy of the event. Birth is the unforeseeable spectacle[12] she had been involved in. In order to succeed in "giving birth to a healthy child" Samia had to cooperate and to expose herself. Samia had witnessed herself having been "handed off [weitergereicht]" and having done what she was told.

I would like to describe Samia's perception of having been unsheathed as a state of *existential nakedness* (Janz 2011, p. 465)[13]: Samia felt ashamed because she was corporeally and existentially naked and was neither able to cover herself nor escape from herself.[14] Being existentially naked means being aware of oneself while being in a kind of oblivion of oneself (Janz 2011, p. 465).[15] This alienating experience could be described in terms of eye-witnessing. Eye-witnessing as an analytic term stresses the existential nakedness interpreted in the sense of hierarchy and power differences. Being eye-witnessed signifies being exposed to someone else's and to one's own observation at the same time. So eye-witnessing describes a double witnessing.

Samia obviously doubted her "scope of action", her own involvement in giving birth. She told the midwife that she, the midwife, would have been the one who had given birth to her child. "No, it has been only you", the midwife reassured her and Samia seemed to be very happy about it. The midwife seemed to really mean it, Samia told me: "I could see it in her eyes". Interestingly, the "cold" eyes she had been exposed to transmitted trustworthiness as well. This multiple and paradoxical potential of witnessing is one of its characteristic features: Samia had seen herself being exposed to the clinical management of her *body-in-labour*. She had been alienated to a degree that made her doubt her proper participation in giving birth to her child. The midwife is responding to Samia's need with the same eyes—not cold anymore, but warm and friendly—which unsheathed Samia during birth. In order to reconnect with her exposure Samia charges the midwife to re-establish her scope of action for her.

Apart from seeing and speaking, touching is a significant technique in witnessing in midwifery practice. Of course, touching is not *only* witnessing, but also doing something practical. As I mentioned before: putting hands on is an active intervention. Anyhow, in certain situations touching can be understood as an active production of testimonials. These testimonials differ depending on how, where and why they are performed.

Touching as a Witnessing Strategy

The core element of what is called the midwifery craftwork or the midwifery art is body work. Body work is leading from bodies and directed at bodies (Twigg 2006; Twigg et al. 2011). Body work includes professional competences such as observation, developing and using tacit knowledge and performed knowledge (Hirschauer 2008) and applying certain—for instance, labour- and birth-facilitating—postures, gestures or procedures. Several important examinations for surveying the growth and the condition of the child or the condition of the mother are performed with the help of intimate touches. These touches can be realized in more or less caring manners and are not purely instrumental per se. Touch can be imposed: "I have to examine you", or it can be proposed: "Do you want me to examine you?"; "Should we have a look at how it went?". Touch can be a medium of creating a contact between mother, midwife and the unborn child: Midwife while touching the mother's womb: "Hello child, how are you? Oh, you are awake?" and to the mother: "For how long has he been awake this morning?" or it can happen silently, routinely, en passant. In any case, these touches intentionally lead to a diagnostic or therapeutic result. They are testifying the position of the foetus, its existence even. In doing so, they are creating medically and legally relevant testimonials. But they create social and cultural testimonial as well. The midwife testifies certain traits (liveliness, laziness), gender (shy girl, strong boy) or the mother-child-relationship ("Where do you feel the baby kick?") as well. Touching is always a strong intervention and it depends on its qualities and aims if it creates or intensifies alienation directed to the touched body or if it intensifies or re-establishes the association of body and self (Akrich and Pasveer 2004, p. 64). If touch supports association processes, it is to be performed within the woman's scope of action: the woman is explicitly and honestly agreeing to be touched or she is asking for the touch herself, but also the midwife's scope of action: time and a trustful, continual relationship permit a participative and perceptive presence.

When I arrived at the birthplace late in the evening, Jasmin was taking a bath. The midwife and a friend were sitting next to her. It was very warm and sticky in the small and sparely lit bathroom. Jasmin laughed and talked a lot until contractions became heavier. The midwife praised Jasmin after each contraction: "Great! You are doing great!" She proposed that Jasmin change position when she said she felt a "pressing pain". Jasmin was kneeling and saying that the contraction she was having would not end. Via the Doppler foetal monitor the midwife used, we could hear the heartbeat of the child beating slower and slower. Impressively calm, the midwife administered Jasmin with medication, ceasing the contraction. The child's heart regained its rhythm. Jasmin was unrecognizable: distracted and carried away. She turned to her midwife: "I was afraid just now. Could you caress me? Could you breathe with me?" The midwife sat next to her and Jasmin fell into her arms.

As well as Samia and Katharina, Jasmin felt alienated and even threatened by her body-in-labour. She asked the midwife to caress with her and breathe with her so that she could "re-corporate". Witnessing as a perceptive and participatory presence can also be carried out by touch. This presence transmitted by touch can be a source of (re-)association of body and self. Touch as an intimate intervention is associated with trust. When being touched by midwives, women have to trust that midwives know what they are doing and that their touches are skilful and respectful.

Trust as a Strategy of Being Witnessed

"Trust" or even "basic trust" seems to be a leitmotif, a grounding feature of the relationship between pregnant and childbearing women and midwives. Firstly, midwives seem to have a kind of credit of trust. During my participant observation I always experienced that at the very moment I told women and families that I am a midwife, they open their doors for me even though I am a stranger. When we had seen each other several times, they sometimes asked me what my research will be about, even though I had told them when we met first. What I was actually doing seemed less important than the fact that I am a midwife. A midwife's presence nearby a pregnant or childbearing woman seems to be self-evident. Secondly, trust is intensified in bodily interaction and in relation to the degree of intimacy. Thirdly, trust is a strategy to handle potentially shaming and even molesting situations.[16]

Helma had been attended by the same midwife during both of her pregnancies, births and postpartum stages. She told me about the "basic trust" she would have for her midwife and the midwife would have for her. So I asked her what the midwife did that lets her, Helma, be this confident. Apparently it is more important what Helma herself does in order to establish and maintain a trustful relationship: "I open up completely. But I didn't have any problems with it from the beginning on. You lay down and you are examined [vaginally]. Somehow this is the most normal thing in the world. And that, I think, is so nice".

Helma describes trust and her capacity to abandonment relating to the midwife in the context of intimate physical interventions. Being examined vaginally out of an explicitly sexual context in agreement with all interactors is just not "the most normal thing in the world". It seems to be the intimate intervention which "opens up Helma completely". Helma legitimizes the vaginal examination by trusting and by perceiving it as being "the most normal thing in the world". Samia described it very similarly: "I would say the head was turned off, one simply did what was said, because then one had confidence, too, and one knew that one was in good hands and at the end comes the child". Being trustful is also a legitimizing consequence of handing over responsibility to the midwife. Samia is following advice in order to achieve a purpose, which is giving birth to her child. Being trustful seems to be without any alternative.

Finally, women expect to have an intensive and trustful relationship with the midwife as Dörte explained:

> And that I know somehow for this period I can build up a very intensive relationship. Not only in prenatal and postnatal care but also that in the middle so to speak. That self-indulgence and intimacy somehow. And

> nevertheless dealing professionally with each other. This extreme opening-up-to-each-other and just letting yourself go. I still find quite impressive. It starts with somehow being able to say all you want without feeling embarrassed. And during birth this self-indulgence and intimacy. Somehow just letting yourself go. This is definitely special.

As well as Samia and Helma, Dörte describes a trustful relationship as one in which she does not feel embarrassed or in which she is anticipating shame by trusting. Trust is intimately linked to the inevitability of bodily exposure during childbirth, pregnancy and antenatal care. In order get along with "this extreme opening-up-to-each-other", "letting yourself go", are required strategies within a professional relationship. Dörte defines professionalism as being able to say and do things in interaction with her midwife without fearing consequences. Dörte calls it the "objective gaze [den objektiven Blick]"[17]: She can speak to her midwife about difficulties in the relationship to her husband without worrying her midwife "developing an opinion" about her husband as friends or family members would. Objectivity as a feature of the witnessing role does not exclude intimacy per se and does not necessarily lead to alienation. Witnessing objectively means to be an intimate part of a situation without being durably involved. Temporal and local limitations seem to be important variables of witnessing in midwifery care.

Technological Testifying

Finally, I would like to show that technical devices produce powerful testimonials in midwifery care. One of them is the CTG,[18] which has advanced to be one of the obstetrics' and midwife's assistants.

In hospitals, CTGs are usually permanently located next to the head side of a bed replacing the bedside table. Often women have to stay next to it, because cables join the sonic heads to the device. During birth in clinical settings it is used regularly, even continuously. In birthplaces or at women's homes they are replaced by much smaller Doppler foetal monitors or a wooden ear trumpet called the Pinard horn. In hospitals as well as in birthplaces, CTGs often seem to replace the absent midwife, even though it is "only" registering the foetal heartbeat.

I accompanied Agnes on a visit to Ruth. Ruth attended her fourth child and the birthing date had already passed. Ruth had had two of her three children at home with Agnes. Agnes visited her regularly now in order to register the foetal heartbeat, verifying if the baby is still going well. Agnes announced she would register for ten minutes only, because it would be no more than a "snapshot" anyway. While Ruth lay down on her sofa, Agnes installed the device in front of which she was kneeling on the floor. The CTG's tone was set off, but both of them stopped talking and fixed the paper with the two jagged lines gliding out. A midwife's witnessing expertise is established with the help of the CTG. It produces a public and durable artefact which serves as a testimonial. This artefact testifies the foetus's vitality without penetrating the mother's body. Like ultrasound, it creates something visible out of something invisible. It seems to extend the witnessing-room of the midwife, but actually it creates its own witnessing presence. The testimony it bears or produces is material and supposedly objective, which the midwife is not able to do. Agnes emphasizes the fugitive character of the CTG to try to diminish its competitive significance, even though both Agnes and Ruth are subjected to its presence. In hospital, midwives do not seem to compete with the CTG, but co-operate and even subordinate. In this setting, the CTG is a potent producer of testimonials because of its objectivity, materiality, continuity and its impetus-giving character.[19] Therefore, it fulfils the legal criteria of witnessing. The presence of CTGs is helpful when midwives attend several women at once in clinical settings, which usually happens. In this case, the midwives as well as women in labour usually seem to feel more secure as a result of the CTG's continual presence and surveillance of the child. But the CTG certainly also affords frequent absences of midwives and doctors by surveilling mother and child.

Conclusion: Witnessing Configurations in Midwifery Care

I introduced witnessing as a mode of being-with of midwives and women during pregnancy, birth and the postpartum stage. I pointed out that witnessing as it is idealized in the legal context, but also in certain philosophical traditions does not work out. As the witness is embodied, she is not neutral but involved in situations and related to people, surroundings, and things. I used witnessing characteristics as being more passive and receptive than active, being knowledgeable, being trustable and being a witness because of having been assigned to be a witness to describe midwifery care. Witnessing is not the only mode of action and interaction concerning midwives and women, of course. It has its limits: Witnessing ends if hands-on action leaves no room for passivity, for passive activeness as I called it. Witnessing cannot happen if women do not assume their body: their body-in-labour, their dys-appearing body, and want to escape and leave it to the midwife. Witnessing always involves a distance. Even if one and the same person is witnessing herself, which results from and leads to alienating experiences, there is distance involved. Women handle the shaming potential of being witnessed bodily exposed—I called it eye-witnessing—by trusting the midwife not only in advance but also in reaction. Witnessing seems to be easier when there are fewer temporal and structural restraints. In clinical settings, witnessing is a lot more difficult and eye-witnessing is more likely. How to witness if it is impossible to stay nearby the woman because several women at once have to be attended to? How to witness if guidelines and standards impose certain medical interventions? Apparently, midwives' scope of action and women's scope of action are entangled with each other. It would be helpful to create environments in which midwives-women relationships happen which give opportunity to midwives to have time and space to attend one woman continually, even at the hospital, and which give opportunity to women to be involved in decision-making and action-taking and to be carefully protected against exposure (see also Hodnett et al. 2013; Sandall et al. 2013).

Acknowledgements I would like to thank Annelieke Driessen, Tim Opgenhaffen, Kristine Krause, Jeannette Pols, Theresa Kerbusk, Tanja Müller and Franziska Krause for their helpful comments on previous drafts of this paper.

Notes

1. I understand embodiment as a corporeal bounded, interacting and interactive being-in-the-world. The phenomenological description of the body (the German *Leib*) as the condition of experience and concernment as well as the sociological view on how bodies are constructed or shaped (*doing bodies*) are part of this embodiment.

2. How uncomfortable this disembodied state might be is marvellously illustrated by Roald Dahl in his short story *William and Mary* (Dahl 2004).
3. In legal contexts, witnessing and testifying are spatially and temporally separated. In contrast, I would suggest there is simultaneity of witnessing and testifying in space and time in midwifery care (apart from the paper work which serves as testimonial and can be defined as a legal act).
4. According to the *Hebammengesetz* (1985/2014), midwives are supposed to *survey* [überwachen] birth, provide intrapartum assistance and *survey* postpartum stage. Surveillance entails control and distance within a hierarchical structure. Witnessing could be described as a "soft" surveillance which is interrelated, which involves mutual responsibility and trust and within which hierarchies as well as distance and proximity are constantly shifting.
5. In this article, I draw on observations I made during an internship in southern France and during my midwifery training in Germany as well.
6. Actually this did not seem to happen out of uncertainty, but in order to get to know my point of view. There might have been a certain apprehension about me judging about professional competences or the quality of the provided care. I am even more thankful for having been admitted to observe!
7. I am aware of the fact that midwives are women, too. In midwifery it is totally unusual to talk about women as patients or customers, because midwives usually tend to characterize pregnancy, birth and the postpartum stage as a non-pathological process during which they do not provide service (only) but also care.
8. It would be interesting to spend more thoughts on knitting as a cultural phenomenon. Knitting is a traditional feminine occupation and craftwork belonging to the private sphere. A renaissance of knitting as a social and ecological and therefore even political activity can be stated in western cultures. The act of knitting itself seems to be more important than its products, which is the case for the knitting midwife, too. The knitting midwife belongs to the private sphere and would not be situated in a clinical setting.
9. The French term *sage-femme* for midwife can be translated literally as "wise woman". The English term *midwife* signifies literally "woman who is with". Both terms contain the passive and knowing presence which is also described by the image of the knitting midwife. The German term *Hebamme* has a more practical-active meaning: The "ancestor/grand-

mother who lifts the child (during birth)". Wisdom (usually attributed to the elder) leads to a practical knowing-how.

10. Uterine contractions lead to a progressive opening of the cervix from ca. 1 cm until 10 cm during birth. The first 3 cm of opening take quite a long time—especially if the woman is giving birth for the first time—and this phase is not yet considered as the active phase of labour, but the so-called latent phase.
11. Madeleine Akrich and Bernike Pasveer analysed women's childbirth narratives and concluded that women would differentiate between an embodied self and a *body-in-labour*. I would like to borrow the term *body-in-labour* from Akrich; Pasveer to the extent to which it illustrates externally and internally induced objectification processes during birth which might create a sensation of this *body-in-labour* being separated from the embodied self of the woman in labour (Akrich and Pasveer 2004).
12. I understand "doing circus" as being involved in a spectacle (Lat. spectare: to watch) which means having been watched.
13. In his article, "Shame and silence" the American professor of philosophy Bruno B. Janz develops further a former publication of Samantha Vice (2010). He refers to Emmanuel Levinas and Gorgio Agamben in order to show what "kind of self [...] whiteness in South Africa makes possible today" (Janz 2011, p. 462). Non-white people might evoke an existential shame in white people because of the "immiseration and oppression of blacks during apartheid" (Janz 2011, p. 467). It might seem as if I was using an inadequate template—the midwife-mother relationship is certainly not necessarily comparable to the situation of non-white and white people living together in South Africa—but actually I am borrowing a philosophical anthropological approach to the self in the same way in which Janz is using Agamben's concept of witnessing of Auschwitz survivors (Janz 2011, p. 469).
14. Agamben explains that shame derives from discovering oneself (or one's Being) and not being able to avoid it. Being ashamed also means being aware of oneself (see Agamben 2002).
15. Jean-Paul Sartre has also worked on "le regard d'autrui" (the look of the other), which objectifies and alienates (see for instance: Sartre 1982).
16. Luhmann describes trust as the anticipation of disappointment (cf. Luhmann 2014, p. 104). I would like to argue here that trust is established in practices and has to be constantly renewed. Trust can be a reaction to a disappointing (shaming, frightening, painful etc.) situation as well.

17. Dörte does not use the term "objective gaze" in the Foucauldian sense of the "medical gaze" (Foucault 2011). For her the objective gaze is a relating, but respectfully distant gaze.
18. The CTG records the foetal heart sounds and the uterine contractions during pregnancy and birth. While recording it reproduces the foetal heartbeat laudably and prints out a paper with two curves on scales representing the foetal heartbeat and the maternal contractions.
19. Intrapartum care is usually based on information given by the CTG.

References

Agamben, G. (2002). *Remnants of Auschwitz. The Witness and the Archive*. New York: Zone Books.

Akrich, M., & Pasveer, B. (2004). Embodiment and Disembodiment in Childbirth Narratives. *Body & Society, 10*(2–3), 63–84.

Dahl, R. (2004). William and Mary. In R. Dahl (Ed.), *Kiss Kiss* (pp. 19–46). London: Penguin Books.

Derrida, J. (2005). *Poétique et Politique du Témoignage*. Paris: L'Herne.

Drews, W., & Schlie, H. (2011). Zeugnis und Zeugenschaft: Perspektiven aus der Vormoderne. Zur Einleitung. In W. Drews & H. Schlie (Eds.), *Zeugnis und Zeugenschaft: Perspektiven aus der Vormoderne* (pp. 7–21). München: Fink.

Foucault, M. (2011). *Die Geburt der Klinik. Eine Archäologie des ärztlichen Blicks*. Frankfurt am Main: Fischer.

Glaser, Barney G., & Anselm Strauss. (1971). *The Discovery of Grounded Theory. Strategies for Qualitative Research* (4th printing). New York: Aldine.

Hirschauer, S. (2008). Körper macht Wissen: für eine Somatisierung des Wissensbegriffs. In K.-S. Rehberg (Ed.), *Die Natur der Gesellschaft: Verhandlungen des 33. Kongresses der Deutschen Gesellschaft für Soziologie in Kassel 2006* (pp. 974–984). http://www.gesetze-im-internet.de/bundesrecht/hebg_1985/gesamt.pdf. 20 Apr 2016.

Hebammengesetz (HebG). (1985/2014). URL: http://www.gesetze-im-internet.de/bundesrecht/hebg_1985/gesamt.pdf, 20 Apr 2016.

Hodnett, E. D., Gates, S., Hofmeyr, G. J., & Sakala, C. (2013). Continuous Support for Women During Childbirth. *The Cochrane Library*. doi:10.1002/14651858.CD003766.pub5.

Janz, B. B. (2011). Shame and Silence. *South African Journal of Philosophy, 30*(4), 462–471.

Krämer, S. (2011). Vertrauenschenken. Über Ambivalenzen der Zeugenschaft. In S. Schmidt (Ed.), *Politik der Zeugenschaft: zur Kritik einer Wissenspraxis* (pp. 117–140). Bielefeld: Transcript.

Leder, D. (1990). *The Absent Body*. Chicago: University of Chicago Press.

Luhmann, N. (2014). *Vertrauen. Ein Mechanismus der Reduktion sozialer Komplexität*. Konstanz: UVK Verlagsgesellschaft.

Onfray, M. (1992). *Der sinnliche Philosoph: über die Kunst des Genießens*. Frankfurt am Main: Campus.

Sandall, J., Soltani, H., Gates, S., Shennan, A., & Devane, D. (2013). Midwife-Led Continuity Models Versus Other Models of Care for Childbearing Women. *The Cochrane Library*. doi:10.1002/14651858.CD004667.pub3.

Sartre, J.-P. (1982). *Huis clos*. Paris: Gallimard.

Schmidt, S. (2011). Wissensquelle oder ethisch-politische Figur? Zur Synthese zweier Forschungsdiskurse über Zeugenschaft. In S. Schmidt (Ed.), *Politik der Zeugenschaft: zur Kritik einer Wissenspraxis* (pp. 47–66). Bielefeld: Transcript.

Strauss, A. L. (1987). *Qualitative Analysis for Social Scientists*. Cambridge: Cambridge University Press.

Twigg, J. (2006). *The Body in Health and Social Care*. New York: Palgrave Macmillan.

Twigg, J., Wolkowitz, C., Cohen, R. L., & Nettleton, S. (2011). Conceptualising Body Work in Health and Social Care. *Sociology of Health & Illness, 33*(2), 171–188.

Vice, S. (2010). How Do I Live in This Strange Place? *Journal of Social Philosophy, 41*(3), 323–342.

Open Access This chapter is licensed under the terms of the Creative Commons Attribution 4.0 International License (http://creativecommons.org/licenses/by/4.0/), which permits use, sharing, adaptation, distribution and reproduction in any medium or format, as long as you give appropriate credit to the original author(s) and the source, provide a link to the Creative Commons license and indicate if changes were made.

The images or other third party material in this chapter are included in the chapter's Creative Commons license, unless indicated otherwise in a credit line to the material. If material is not included in the chapter's Creative Commons license and your intended use is not permitted by statutory regulation or exceeds the permitted use, you will need to obtain permission directly from the copyright holder.

Tensions in Diabetes Care Practice: Ethical Challenges with a Focus on Nurses in a Home-Based Care Team

Pei-Yi Liu and Helen Kohlen

Introduction

The prevalence of diabetes is rising worldwide and the condition has become a major health and economic problem. Diabetes is a chronic illness which results in a relentless, ongoing and incurable suffering, and an inseparable part of it is the suffering of the whole person. The appropriate management of diabetes care includes more than just glycaemic control. How to support patients to live well with diabetes is a tough lifelong task for both patients and healthcare professionals.

The authors would like to acknowledge the research support of the department of the home-care centre (PflegeNetz) at the university hospital Freiburg, which provided the opportunity to have conversations with the participants on which this study is based.

P.-Y. Liu (✉)
Faculty of Nursing, Philosophisch-Theologische Hochschule Vallendar (PTHV), Vallendar, Germany

H. Kohlen
Lehrstuhl Care Policy und Ethik, Philosophisch-Theologische Hochschule Vallendar (PTHV), Vallendar, Germany

© The Author(s) 2018
F. Krause, J. Boldt (eds.), *Care in Healthcare*,
https://doi.org/10.1007/978-3-319-61291-1_11

Scholars have engaged in promoting the quality of diabetes care for a long time. Disease self-management and self-efficacy have been reported as important concepts in diabetes care and empowering patients to be active can lead to successful diabetes management (Moser et al. 2006; Shigaki et al. 2010). For patients and healthcare professionals, respecting the disease without letting it dominate the patient's life is key (Ingadottir 2009, pp. 77–92). Normalizing the process of managing diabetes can encourage patients to regulate their lifestyles with respect to controlling the disease (Olshansky et al. 2008).

In diabetes care practice, an individual care plan tailoring to the patient's needs and ongoing care provided by healthcare professionals who work together could be suggested as constituting good care (McDonald et al. 2012). A collaborative healthcare team can not only strengthen diabetes self-care in practice, but also ensure that effective medical, preventive and health maintenance interventions take place (Von Korff et al. 1997). The foregoing argumentation reinforces the need for implementation of "The Logic of Care" in diabetes care practice to achieve improvement.

"The Logic of Care" is based on Mol's field research. Using methods such as ethnographic observations, background research and interviews with diabetes patients and medical practitioners in a hospital in the Netherlands, Mol (2008) engaged critically with the current healthcare models which see patients as consumers and citizens. In the light of Mol's argumentation, care is not a limited product, but more like a dynamic and open-ended process (Mol 2008, p. 14). A caring process consists of interactive relationships among all of the caring actors (e.g. patients and professionals), and it can be shifted and adapted according to different care outcomes (Mol 2008, p. 20). With respect to the concept of patients as citizens who have abilities and rights to make their own choices and enact their will, Mol elaborated that the patient-citizens have little choice but to bracket a part of what they are and seek ways to live with a disease (Mol 2008, p. 35). Caring is therefore a matter of being attuned, respecting and being adaptable instead of controlling (Mol 2008, p. 36).

By Mol's assumption, care has its own logic. But one kind of logic (e.g. the logic of care) is not always intrinsically better than other kinds of logic (e.g. the logic of choice) (Mol 2008, p. 92). In practice, we sometimes need the logic of care, but it can be employed alongside other logics depending on the care situation. It is important that all caring actors be active (Mol 2008, p. 93). In this paper, we utilized "The Logic of Care" conceptualized by Mol for our research approach. Meanwhile, we stressed the ethical dilemmas occurring in a home-based care team.

The notion of the global marketplace has spread to the domain of health services, so that health has come to be seen as a commodity, with the body as its site and the patient as a customer (Parker 1999). Patients' satisfaction has become a significant indicator to measure the quality of care when patient-centred care is supplied (Robin et al. 2008; Wagner and Bear 2009).[1] The challenge for healthcare workers is to work within, but also to resist the reductionist impetus of economically based and commercially driven approaches to healthcare (Parker 1999). Healthcare workers face the rigorous tasks of maintaining holistic care, preserving the personal and professional–recipient relationship and finding ways of demonstrating their capacity to deliver high-quality care in a cost-effective way (Parker 1999). Moral tensions may accordingly arise.

Moral tensions in care practice may additionally originate in the different understanding of illness and the distinct demands of diabetes care on healthcare professionals and patients. Patients focus more often on consequences and the impact on their daily life, while healthcare professionals pay more attention to the medical treatment and economic efficiency (Hörnsten et al. 2004). Whereas healthcare professionals pay much attention to the best interests of patients, they usually have to exercise both clinical and moral responsibilities in relation with patients. For this reason, care responsibilities are determined not only by considerations of the patients' rights and respect for their freedom but also by consideration of the wider health needs of the individual and the community (Thompson et al. 2006).

In the healthcare system, medical orientation, hierarchy, authority and unequal power among physicians, patients and nurses are noticeable (Daiski 2004; Kramer and Schmalenberg 2003). The hierarchy between different professionals affects how a professional can act on his own moral position (Kälvemark et al. 2004). How do healthcare workers work within this kind of medical environment and simultaneously preserve their professional awareness? Which care problems and ethical dilemmas can be raised? How do healthcare workers practically reflect on care problems and ethical dilemmas? And how do healthcare workers deal with them in their daily work? To further grasp the ethical dilemmas in diabetes care, it makes sense to take a look at the actors and to review how authority, responsibility and trust play out among physicians, patients and nurses in everyday practice.

Nurses have hitherto played a barely visible role in the German healthcare system, but they have implicitly been expected to fulfil the dominant care role. The nurse is not only the person who provides the care in practice, but also the one who has the most contact with patients and who understands patients better than other healthcare professionals (Rich 2008). We would like to take home-care nurses as an example in this paper to explore how tensions arise and how they are dealt with in the field of patient care.[2]

Methods and Materials

This study is a case study with a qualitative approach. This paper concentrates on home-care nurses' experiences and tensions in diabetes care practice where complex care takes place involving a multi-professional team.

The home-care centre at the university hospital Freiburg in southwest Germany served as the setting for the research case.[3] A field observation and in-depth interviews were implemented to collect empirical data. The interview participants were six home-care nurses who had a diabetes care education or a background of diabetes care experience and had held their current position in the German home-care context for at least two years.

From April to November 2012, direct and participant observations and structured face-to-face interviews with home-care nurses took place. Narrative thematic interviews were performed using an interview guide covering topics related to the experience in diabetes management, the experience of multi-professional team work and needs in diabetes care.[4]

Interviews and feedback sessions were audiotaped and transcribed verbatim for the thematic analysis of the content. Some selected transcripts of interviews were coded by a research group to identify additional insights. Data management was facilitated by the use of a computer program (NVivo 10). The analysis of the interviews was guided by Creswell's thematic analysis (2007, pp. 147–176). A two-level coding scheme was used, starting with a provisional list of codes based on selected concepts identified in the literature, with new codes added based on the data (Miles et al. 2013). In an iterative process of coding and condensing the data, recurring themes emerged. In terms of an ethical scheme, three abstracted themes were identified as underlying or latent messages in diabetes care practice; these were then confirmed as being common to all categories.

Findings

By analysing the empirical data focused on the experience of home-care nurses, three themes emerged: identification of care receivers, performance of care actions and foundations of care relationships. These frame the tensions home-care nurses face while working with patients and with other healthcare professionals in the diabetes care context. The tensions around the three themes are:

- The identification of care receivers: Tension between patients and customers.
- The performance of care actions: Tension between an ongoing process and finding an end by acceptance.
- The foundations of care relationships: Tension between authority and responsibility.

Patients Versus Customers

In diabetes care, home-care nurses stated that they treat their care receivers as patients instead of customers.[5] For nurses, the person who receives medical treatment is considered a patient in the nurse–patient relationship, whether his disease is acute or chronic. This way, nurses are able to provide continuous medical care for outpatients from hospitals to the surrounding where they live. The care relationship ends the day when nurses accept that patients don't want it and hand over the responsibility to them:

> So we call all of our patients 'patients'. So we don't have customers. Because we get most of our patients directly from the hospital and they have been treated as patients there. Therefore, they will also be simply treated as patients by us. I cannot call a part of my patients 'customers' and the other part of them 'patients'. [...] When patients are independent someday, like Mr. Harry, then we can leave them and say that the patient relationship is closed. But as long as we take care of a patient, he is a patient for us. He won't be a customer sometimes only because of his chronic disease. (I-NN-01)

When nurses talked about good care, it meant that all of the patients, nurses and physicians feel satisfied with their care outcome. A good care outcome for diabetes care was quickly linked to good blood sugar values: "For me, good care means simply that the patient is satisfied, we are satisfied and the family doctor is satisfied with the blood sugar values" (I-NN-01).

In care practice, nurses avoided to challenge patients' autonomy and respected their right to choose the way they live. Nurses think that they can't force patients to act, but can only offer suggestions.[6] However, offering suggestions doesn't always lead to success:

> I can't force anybody to do anything. I can only suggest to them to do things which are good for their bodies and I can always try to say, 'You should move more often', but it doesn't always work. (I-NN-05)

An Ongoing Process Versus Finding an End by Acceptance

Nurses recognized that creating fear and exerting control is not a good idea for diabetes care. They said, "We are not there to control" (I-NN-01). Indeed, nurses cannot control what their patients eat or what they do throughout the day since they only come for a short visit. Instead of controlling, it is more important to offer an alternative way of keeping in touch with patients. However, attempts to work with alternatives have run into difficulties in practice. Eight minutes are planned in the schedule for one home-visit with a diabetes patient. The time pressure and insufficient knowledge limit nurses' work a lot. In particular, nurses have no chance to try alternatives if their patients reject their advice:

> It would be very good if we could take more care of diabetes patients, including offering advice on nutrition. But we have no time, and in many cases we don't have current knowledge. We simply don't have enough knowledge on nutrition counselling. And some patients do not want it either. They reject it. (I-NN-04)

Nurses expressed that continually trying to achieve their care goals is their wish as a healthcare professional, and a few nurses believed that "constant dripping wears the stone" (I-NN-06). Unfortunately, patients' lack of intention to follow up on the principles of diabetes management restrains nurses from going further during the care process. In the following case, a nurse tried to motivate her patients at the beginning, but after some failed attempts, the nurse eventually accepted her patient's decision even though this decision was against her will. However, this outcome led to an uncomfortable feeling on the part of the nurse and hurt the patient–nurse relationship as well:

> The patient was exasperated one day and told me, 'Stop now, I don't want to hear about it [diabetes care] any more'. Then I said, 'Okay, let's let it go'. Then I said nothing about it any more. I had argued with him because of his diabetes. But he still eats chocolate, doesn't change his life. Then he has to inject more and more Insulin and is getting fatter. He wants that. One day you have to say, 'Okay' and accept it. Although it is a difficult decision, but what should I do? I cannot beat him and push him on the way, right. (I-NN-06)

The tension, however, creates a lot of stress for nurses when they have to accept undesired outcomes. Nurses feel pity and are disappoint about situations in which improvements cannot be made: "This is of course an example in which one has a bad feeling. At this point, you will ask yourself about what you still expect" (I-NN-03). Sometimes, nurses face critical care situations without the possibility of making a difference. Nurses then have to deal with feelings of fear and guilt:

> It happened often that his blood sugar values were 18 mg/dl or something like that. That's a very, very uncomfortable situation. And I have faced such tense situations twice. That's a very unsettling and scary situation. But as I said, it cannot be changed. (I-NN-01)

Authority Versus Responsibility

In home-care practice, nurses usually identify as mediators vis-à-vis the healthcare team and see themselves as advocates for the patients. Nurses reported that their mission in practice is to create a bridge between physicians and patients:

> We can actually only play the role of a mediator or a messenger when, for instance, the patient has difficulties to communicate with his family doctor or when the family doctor doesn't visit his patient regularly. Then we have to call the doctor and inform him, 'The patient's values are not good and we need to do something to change it'. In this case, we play the role of an advocate for the patient. So we are simply mediators and advocates. (I-NN-01)

Good cooperative teamwork is important for healthcare, but not always seen in practice. Information flows are often interrupted in a variety of ways between different medical organizations. In practice, home-care nurses often receive a medical plan without the related background. This is neither a satisfying nor a safe situation for nurses. For one thing, nurses are then unsure about their work. In addition, they cannot explain changes in their care to the patients. Nurses have pointed out that they have to take responsibility for the care they offer, and that they therefore want to get clear answers. Nevertheless, they are sometimes too fearful to clarify their questions with physicians because of the strict hierarchy and the nurses' low position in the current healthcare system:

> I would like to know why the doctor raised the Insulin dosage. I'm still not sure what I should do now. Should I contact with the family doctor or a diabetes specialist? Should I send a fax to the family doctor and ask him why he has raised the dosage? But I think that sending a fax is so impersonal. I do not know him. Maybe he will feel that I am stepping on his toes if I, as a 'lowly' nurse, ask him something about his medical plan. But I couldn't explain to my patient why he needs more Insulin now, and I was also surprised about it myself. [...] I am not one to merely follow orders. I also have a responsibility for what I do. (I-NN-06)

Many nurses have mentioned that communication with physicians is not always a comfortable experience. Nurses have complained that it is difficult to reach physicians or to talk to them. Sometimes nurses have tried to communicate with physicians via the patients. However, this indirect way may lead to inter-professional mistrust. Furthermore, nurses have sometimes suggested to their patients to change their family physician in order to create a safe care environment and allow for cooperative teamwork:

> When I inform a family doctor that his patient is in a bad condition, then he must respond to my request and do something. [...] If he doesn't act, I will say to the patient, 'It took such a long time until your doctor came. Maybe you should consider taking another doctor who comes quickly'. I have already done that. Whether the patient does it or not is another matter, because patients usually say, 'Oh, we have already had that doctor for 20 years and he has always come'. (I-NN-06)

Many nurses believe that patients' have a lot more trust in their physicians than in nurses. According to the nurses' experience, patients follow what their doctors say, no matter what it is. This creates a tension for nurses. Even if the nurses disagree with the physicians' opinions, they will still obey the physicians' orders. Nurses do so not only because physicians have the legal right to have "the last word", but also because the nurses don't want to confuse patients with two opposing sets of advice:

> What doctors say is right. So even if I sometimes don't agree with what the doctors say, I don't want to confuse my patients. I cannot just go to a

patient and say, 'What a nonsense your doctor told to you', because the patient will become totally uncertain. I have experienced that one time, when I said to the patient, 'We must do that', and the patient answered, 'Oh, but my doctor told me something quite different.' And then he became very uncertain. (I-NN-02)

Discussion[7]

Can Care Receivers Be Both "Customers" and "Patients"?

The first theme of the research interprets the tension regarding the identification of care receivers as customers and patients. According to the research, home-care nurses consider their care receivers "patients" because this helps nurses provide a continuum of care with different organizations. Nevertheless, consumer sovereignty[8] is usually taken into consideration in healthcare. It is reflected in nurses' care activities in that they avoid putting pressure on patients. For instance, when a patient rejects a nurse's offer of a nutrition consultant's services, this approach to care is discontinued in practice. In this case, the logic of choice is at work and the care receiver is treated more like a customer than a patient.

Since consumer sovereignty has high priority in the healthcare market, patients are often practically treated as customers and as citizens and choices are made following the patients' wishes (Ryl and Horch 2013). Nurses then have difficulties carrying out interventions against patients' will. As a nurse explained, "I cannot force anybody to do anything" (I-NN-05). Nurses often have to compromise, which may run counter to their professional awareness. While the understanding of care receivers as patients and of the value of the person's wholeness is rooted in the identity of the nursing professional, the way nurses have to act is often contrary to this identity in practice. This contradiction can produce a moral tension in nursing work. It might lead to frustration with the caring process or damage the trust-relationship between nurses and patients. We will discuss these two themes later in the second and third sections.

In home-care practice, satisfaction has been used as the main indicator to decide if good care is offered. The terms "quality in care service" and "patient satisfaction" are often connected and brought on the healthcare agenda (Bostan et al. 2007). Patient satisfaction is derived from the marketing perspective. Patients are the most important clients of health institutions and their satisfaction is hence the main product of health institutions (Torpie 2014). Patient satisfaction has been explained in terms of adding value and creating a service exceeding or meeting patients' expectations (Torpie 2014). However, when healthcare professionals only focus on patients' satisfactions during a care process, they provide their services often as commodities according to the customers' desires (Mol 2008, p. 28).

There is a danger in thinking of care as a commodity, as a service for purchase. First, the diverse care goals and needs patients and nurses have may result in a tension for nurses. This is because patients place a lot of trust in those who care for them and for nurses to respond in a trustworthy way, they must care about their patients, not just for them (De Raeve 2002; Hörnsten et al. 2004). Second, when healthcare professionals begin to talk in terms of commodification, they too quickly begin to slip into thinking of the time and cost for a service instead of the needs of those cared for (Olshansky et al. 2008; Tronto 2010). Third, caring for patients is a kind of caritas. Caring for ill people is valuable and meaningful in and of itself and cannot be calculated and priced as a commodity (Maio 2009).

In the words of Duttweiler (2007), health is not a product that can be sold and a patient is not a customer who buys a product, but a person who needs professionals' help to deal with his diseases. In this sense, care professionals have a duty to ensure that patients are able to give their agreement to the care process by, for instance, ensuring their empowerment, which is considered a transformative way of autonomy (Duttweiler 2007). Thus, thinking of care receivers as patients doesn't mean ignoring their autonomy or denying their rights to make decisions about their needs, but providing alternatives, sources of legitimacy and information as counter-acting forces (Tronto 2010).

To take care of patients' satisfaction, to respect patients' rights of make their own choices or to empower patients are different ways of caring.

The concern in diabetes care is not which one is better, but which one is more appropriate to a situation and what can be done in practice (Mol 2008, p. 92). That means that patients' satisfaction can be one of the indicators to measure the quality of care, but it shouldn't be the only one. Consumer sovereignty should be respected, but all of the patients' expectations should not necessarily be fulfilled in practice without thinking of the actual needs for care, especially when dealing with diabetes.

Can "Finding an End" Be Acceptable in an Ongoing Care Process?

The second theme summarized from the research findings is around care actions. Within the logic of care, care is an interactive, open-ended process that may be shaped and reshaped depending on its results (Mol 2008, p. 23). Nevertheless, nursing care has its boundaries in practice. In the research, a tension emerged between continually trying for care improvements and finding an end by accepting an undesired care outcome.

This kind of distress is usually connected with the differences in care goals between patients and nurses, as well as their different perspectives on what "good" is. A care intervention such as asking patients to follow strict nutrition rules may be considered as good for diabetes management, but may limit patients' day-to-day life and happiness a lot. Patients may therefore reject an approach to care during a care process. The logic of care implies the need to pay attention to the information obtained from care practice without passing judgment as to what is good or bad, so that healthcare professionals and patients respect each others' experience and are attuned to each others' strengths and limitations (Mol 2008, p. 65).

While healthcare professionals are carrying out their duty of ensuring patients' safety and devoting themselves to keeping risk and harm away from patients' bodies, patients' wishes and/or desires may often be ignored. For instance, if a nurse tries to prohibit her patient from eating chocolate, which is his favourite food, that patient may suffer from the feeling of being controlled. On the contrary, if the nurse knows more about the background of her patient, she may be able to understand better why the patient takes a given care decision and why the decision is important for him.[9] If nurses can, in their care, balance the priorities and concerns of both patients and healthcare professionals and find a common denominator leading to an outcome in which the patient's safety is ensured, nurses may accept that letting it go can, in some cases, be the best option for a patient, even it doesn't meet the nurses' expectation of the care process. As Mol explained, "The logic of care is not preoccupied with our will, and what we may opt for, but concentrates on what we do". (Mol 2008, p. 8) Unfortunately, nurses do not, in practice, have the time to get all the relevant information or the space and ability to reflect on these kinds of dilemmas in care during their busy and stressful work.

Modifying one's lifestyle is part of diabetes treatment, but it is the most difficult part of diabetes management. In the practice of care, the patients' intentions to follow through on a care intervention influence the care professionals' motivation as well. It is often seen in diabetes care that nurses stop trying to offer a care improvement (e.g. a nutrition consultation) if they recognize that their patients have no interest in it. Likewise, when patients show the will to take part in care activities, nurses do more for them. Yet, a clinician–patient relationship requires more than a customer service oriented by customers' decisions. It is a therapeutic relationship which focuses on caring for an individual more than on customer service (Torpie 2014). In other words, it is sometimes necessary in care practice to push patients to do things for their bodies, just like a diabetes patient must inject insulin regularly if they want to stay alive (Mol 2008, p. 45).

Encouraging patients to be active by sharing doctoring and care responsibility with other care professionals is advisable in diabetes care (Duttweiler 2007; Mol 2008, p. 65). From this point of view, it is important that patients, as customers in the medical market, have to realize their limitations in professional care, to trust their care professionals and to accept help (Duttweiler 2007). Patients have to be educated about their disease and to act themselves during their disease management. Care professionals have to provide support until patients get a full understanding of their disease management and are able to integrate it into their life (Maio 2009; Raspe 1999). It is a long-term process which costs time, money and manpower. When working within a medical care system organized on the basis of economic efficiency, it is unfortunately difficult to bring theory into practice. As a nurse told us, “It would be very good if we could take more care of diabetes patients. […] But we have no time, and in many cases, we don’t have current knowledge. […] And some patients do not want it either. They reject it” (I-NN-03).

Accepting an undesired care outcome is symptomatic for an ambivalence to their professional awareness for home-care nurses and leads to feelings of uncertainty and disappointment. As a nurse said, “ […] at this time, you will ask yourself what you still expect” (I-NN-03). In keeping with their professional identity, nurses expect that a care improvement can be implemented and patients’ safety can be ensured. In reality, nurses can have to deal with critical care situations without any possibility of changing the situation. Nurses might therefore fall into a kind of moral distress, doubting themselves and feeling fear and guilt. During nurses’ daily work, especially in home-based care practice, nurses have only few opportunities to exchange their experiences in care with their care team or to discuss ethical dilemmas with others.

ANA (2008) noted in the “ANA Nursing Code of Ethics”[10]: “The nurse owes the same duties to self as to others, including the responsibility to preserve integrity and safety, to maintain competence, and to continue personal and professional growth”. The research data reflected the requirement to enhance nurses’ personal and professional growth. The “Code of Ethics” further articulated: “Nurses are required to have knowledge relevant to the current scope and standards of nursing practice, changing issues, concerns, controversies and ethics. Where care required is outside the competencies of the individual nurse, consultation should be sought or the patient should be referred to others for appropriate care” (ANA 2008). The logic of care states a similar aspect: “A care process involves a team and tasks are divided between the members of that team in ever-changing ways” (Mol 2008, p. 21). It is essential to develop efficient networking among different care professionals in diabetes care practice. Meanwhile, each care professional has to learn how to work together with other care professionals and has to rethink collaborative ways of working within a team.

Can Care Responsibility Play Out Within Trust-Relationships Without Authority?

This is the third theme associated with the foundations of care relationships. In this section, trust in a nurse–physician relationship and in a nurse–patient relationship is embedded within a healthcare environment full of a sense of responsibility without authority while professional care responsibilities are not made explicit.

The phrase of "responsibility without authority" has been widely used in various scholarly discussions such as social, economic, management, political, medical and healthcare discourses. It often designates the tension in relationships part of a hierarchy, for instance, in a nurse–doctor relationship (Burston and Tuckett 2013; Pendry 2007; Pullon 2008). While analysing the research data and reviewing the literature, it became clear that the expression "responsibility without authority" appeared within the relationships among physicians, nurses and patients in home-based diabetes care practice. While nurses are expected to be responsible for their work, they often experience powerlessness to act within the hierarchical healthcare system where physicians have both the authority and the patients' trust.

In the German healthcare system, medicine is considered as powerful and medical care is seen as a professional endeavour in care practice. The centralization of medical care in society causes an uneven power distribution in professional relationships. Physicians have the power to take medical decisions and nurses have the responsibility to implement them. A moral dilemma can appear in the hierarchy between different professionals when a person who is lower in the hierarchy has to carry out orders from a superior against their own conviction (Kälvemark et al. 2004). Burston and Tuckett (2013) have illustrated how nurses suffer from this care dilemma as "nurses [are] faced with the choice of either overstepping the boundary and acting, or waiting for the physician, watching the suffering of their patients". The problem in this relationship may stem from the different approaches to healthcare delivery, such as a curative as opposed to a care-based approach (Burston and Tuckett 2013).

Traditionally, physicians have authority in medical care and patients trust their physicians as well. A nurse described how she experienced physicians' authority during her daily work in that "what doctors say is right. So even if I sometimes don't agree with what the doctors say, I don't want to confuse my patients" (I-NN-02). This quote reveals how authority, responsibility and trust play out in a care team: The patient trusts his physician; the nurse recognizes what doctors say may not always be right; the nurse experiences difficulties in influencing the decision of her patient; the nurse admits that physicians have the right to have the last word; the nurse knows that she has to be responsible for what she does; the nurse might communicate with the physician or she might be not; the nurse consequently follows the doctor's orders. The care responsibility seems to be silently transferred from one hand to another when the nurse thinks that physicians are in charge. Actually, nurses still have to take responsibility for the care implementation and patients have the right to be informed. Physicians also have to take responsibility for ensuring the safety of medical care. From the above case, we can also observe that physicians' authority invisibly exists within a nurse–patient relationship. Even on the scene, where physicians are not present in a care activity, their authority affects the interactions between nurses and patients.

Another nurse highlights how she is under the physicians' authority in that, "Maybe he (a family doctor) feels his toes are being stepped on if I, as a 'lowly' nurse, ask him something about his medical plan" (I-NN-06). According to the research data, nurses feel dissatisfied and uncertain when communication within a care team is not flowing, when their voices are not heard or not accepted, or when they don't have the authority to negotiate within a care team. Pendry (2007) affirmed that nurses have to carry a lot of responsibility, but lack the necessary executive authority to do anything about a situation. From nurses' point of view, some of the most painful practical tensions arise because they lack the authority to act on their own, to exercise their own judgment, to take the initiative and to go against physicians' orders (Thompson et al. 2006). An international study demonstrated similar findings: "Nurses felt that they lacked either power to speak against physicians' opinions", or "[n]urses believed that their opinions would not be accepted" (Malloy et al. 2009).

To hand over the care responsibility or to accept an undesired care outcome are not pleasant experiences for nurses. Nurses usually feel mistrust and disappointment about themselves, and sometimes about physicians and/or the healthcare system. This tension, as Burston and Tuckett (2013) have articulated, may not only manifest internally or externally, but may harm the individual, others and/or the system. It may further induce feelings of anger towards oneself, self-doubt, diminished self-esteem, depression and even burnout and feelings of anger, bitterness, dismay and frustration towards others (Burston and Tuckett 2013).

An approach whereby all care team members, including physicians, nurses and patients, share the doctoring and the responsibility may help in dealing with this kind of tension in practice. That way, when nurses recognize that physicians are unable to make an optimal decision for a given care situation, nurses would be able to communicate with physicians, enabling them to better take responsibility for the patients' safety. The relevant professional care competencies should be taught in nursing courses and in practice in the field. Physicians also have a responsibility to enhance their professional competencies, including by creating an intensive networking with other healthcare professionals to share doctoring. Additionally, healthcare institutes should be able to organize better cooperative teamwork so that an open and effective dialog among multiple professionals can take place.

Can Professional Identity and Care Competencies Support Trust-Relationships?

Trust toward other professionals as well as towards patients directly and indirectly influences healthcare workers' motivation in providing care (Okello and Gilson 2015). The research indicates that nurses sustain relationships of mistrust with physicians and patients. This originates in the hierarchal medical society, the institutional organization and the care legislation. Nonetheless, nurses' limited professional identity and insufficient professional care competencies are revealed as additional reasons which may frustrate communication with a care team and may further lead to mistrust between nurses, physicians and patients.

Pullon (2008) articulated that the identification and separation of vocational and business roles and the development of a professional identity form the basis for the development of trust in the nurse–physician relationship. In home-care practice, nurses identified their professional roles as mediators and advocates in diabetes care. These two roles are indispensable in the home-based care context because they support inter-professionalism as a platform for the exchange of information. Some studies hold the same point of view and reason that nurses and patients have a closer relationship compared to other healthcare professionals because nursing care occupies an "in between" position in the organization of the public response to the patients' needs. Nurses act to follow up and address their needs appropriately (Rich 2008). Nurses' role as mediators means not only delivering messages from patients to physicians; it consists of the missions to create efficient communication, to share care plans and to identify problems to the care team. Likewise, nurses' role as advocates involves conveying patients' needs in meaningful ways. That is to say that nurses should not only be able to protect patients' rights when something goes wrong, but should also be able to establish a nourishing and safe caring environment. These expanded missions have to be taken into account when we talk about "good care" in home-based diabetes management.

Following Pullon's argumentation, (2008) "[p]rofessional identity is related to the demonstration of professional competence, in turn it is related to the development of mutual inter-professional respect and enduring inter-professional trust". Nurses' professional competencies influence inter-professional trust and patients' trust as well. On the basis of the research data, unequal trust-relationships between patients, nurses and physicians can be observed in home-care practice. Rørtveit and her colleagues (2015) explained that patients' trust in nursing is dependent on the nurses' knowledge, on their level of commitment to dialogue and to creating and developing the relationship and on contextual issues. Yet, the research conveyed a message that nurses are becoming aware of their insufficient knowledge and care competencies in diabetes care. Smith (2012) identified that, "[a]ntecedents to personal and external motivations include the attribution of and integrating of knowledge into practice, experience, critical thinking, proficient skills, caring, communication, environment, motivation, and professionalism". According to his argumentation, issues such as confidence, safe practice and holistic care belong to the caring competencies as well (Smith 2012). In the current healthcare environment, nurses are too overwhelmed to develop the expected competencies and meet the expanded professional roles.

Responding to the argumentation by Maio (2009, p. 32), "[o]ne big problem in modern medical care is that healthcare workers are not reflecting and not able to think about themselves, their identity and the reason why they provide care" (Ein großes Problem der modernen Medizin ist somit ihre Unreflektiertheit, ihre Unfähigkeit, über sich selbst, über ihren Ursprung, über ihre Identität nachzudenken). Encouraging nurses to face ethical dilemmas and to reflect on their nursing work is getting more and more important in care practice. Improving the theoretical and practical training in diabetes care during nursing training and further education programmes may offer a possibility of change. A nourished nursing practice has to be established, wherein nurses have time and space to keep trying to achieve improvements in care. Well-structured institutional regulations for diabetes care may additionally offer legal support for nursing work.[11] It is also necessary to encourage nurses to get a clear understanding of external influences related to nursing education, health legislation and health policy. As Tronto (2010) advocated to healthcare professionals, "recognition and debate/dialogue of relations of power within and outside the organization of competitive and dominative power and agreement of common purpose" should allow nurses not only to recognize the ethical tensions raised in care practice and to learn to reflect on them but also to be able to push a dialogue with the healthcare team, the healthcare system and society. There will be new roles for nurses to grow into and to fill in their practice.

Conclusion

Nurses work within a healthcare system oriented towards economic efficiency. Nurses are, on the one hand, limited by the business approach of serving "customers" and, on the other hand, motivated by the professional awareness of offering medical care for "patients". Nurses attempt to provide patients' with care regulated by their professional identity while satisfying customers' expectations that are dominating the healthcare market. When customer sovereignty and patients' autonomy are emphasized, nurses often have to accept a compromise against their own will. The nursing professional awareness hardly translates into care practice and ethical dilemmas may therefore occur.

Within the hierarchical German medical care system, nurses experience responsibility without authority in the care field. Without authority, nurses find it difficult to engage in teamwork while they are carrying out care responsibilities. Relationships of mistrust towards the care team also come with this. Additional reasons arise from limited professional care competencies and a narrow professional identity. Nurses are overwhelmed in diabetes care, especially in dealing with ethical tensions. To improve personal and professional growth for all healthcare workers and to enhance patients' engagement in disease management is essential. It is also important to create a nourishing and safe care environment wherein professional awareness can be encouraged and acted upon by sharing doctoring and responsibility. The insights gained through this research may assist nurses and other healthcare professionals in reflecting on home-based care teamwork and improving diabetes care in general.

Notes

1. Robin and his colleagues (2008) indicated that patient-centered care (PCC) promotes adherence and leads to improved health outcomes. The fundamental characteristics of PCC were identified as patient involvement in care and the individualization of patient care. Effective PCC practices were related to communication, shared decision making and patient education. However, our research findings showed that an effective PCC is difficult to carry out in practice because of the commercial healthcare market, insufficient competencies on the part of nurses and the hierarchy that arises when patients' satisfaction is used as the indicator to measure the quality of care.
2. Our research does not aim to measure the ethical competencies of healthcare workers or to resolve the ethical tensions that deeply affect the hierarchy. The purpose of this paper is to offer support for healthcare

workers to get a better understanding of the ethical tensions in diabetes care by reflecting on the interactions within a healthcare team, as well as enhancing the sensibility of healthcare workers towards these tensions and inspiring them to think about what can be done in care practice.

3. The Ethics Committee of the University Hospital Freiburg (EK-Freiburg 43/12) approved the study and the participants received the usual assurance about anonymity, confidentially and the right to withdraw at any point.
4. Research questions were asked like: "Can you tell me how you experience caring for patients with diabetes?"; "How do you experience working together with other healthcare professionals such as physicians?"; "Can you tell me an example of how you have reacted to a conflict in care practice?" and "Can you describe what good diabetes care is for you?"
5. The German healthcare is organized as a 'Third Party Payer System'. Patients don't pay healthcare providers directly for their medical treatment within this healthcare system. The healthcare providers calculate the cost of medical services and then receive payments from healthcare insurance (Tscheulin and Dietrich 2010). Thus, patients have a customer status in relation to the health insurance as well as to the service provider, but their "needs" have been considered more often than their "demands" (Raspe 1999; Tscheulin and Dietrich 2010). Nursing care has been talked about as customer care according to the regulations of healthcare insurance as well (Raspe 1999). However, from the perspective of patient care, patients are not customers because their status has been greatly reduced by illness or injury and their sovereignty is therefore limited (Duttweiler 2007; Maio 2009; Raspe 1999; Torpie 2014). It is worth to take a detailed look at how healthcare workers think about their care receivers and how their understanding of care receivers influences their care activities in the field.
6. In the edited volume, "Socio-material will-work", Annelieke Driessen elaborated how healthcare workers applied three kinds of will-work as alternative ways to deal with the wanting of patients to provide good care in the dementia care context.
7. In the discussion part, we draw up some questions formed around tensions to introduce our debate. But our purpose is not to offer clear answers. Instead, we would like to encourage our readers to rethink the tensions based on a variety of discourses. Thus, answers can be different from divergent perspectives, and care work can be presented with a variety of faces.

8. Consumer sovereignty is a phrase often translated as 'the customer is king' and it lays the emphasis on the rights of consumers. Ryl and Horch (2013) indicated that sovereignty is usually presented in healthcare as citizen- and patient-centred care in order to improve the quality of care. In Germany, medical care responds to patients' needs through patient-centred care. In the past ten years, the concept of citizen- and patient-centred care has further developed in the legal and political spheres in the German healthcare system (Ryl and Horch 2013).
9. Björn Freter took a philosophical view of caring for the whole person to discuss the norms for diabetes care. Please see the edited volume (Chapter "Nursing as Accommodated Care. A Contribution to the Phenomenology of Care. Appeal—Concern—Volition—Practice").
10. ANA is the acronym for the American Nurses Association. The Code of Ethics for Nurses was developed as a guide for carrying out nursing responsibilities in a manner consistent with quality in nursing care and the ethical obligations of the profession (ANA 2008).
11. For more on the role of institutional regulation in care, please see the edited volume by Tim Opgenhaffen (Chapter "Regulation as an Obstacle to Care? A Care-Ethical Evaluation of the Regulation on the Use of Seclusion Cells in Psychiatric Care in Flanders (Belgium)") with the legal perspective.

References

American Nurses Association. (2008). Code of Ethics. *Code of Ethics Overview: Provision 5*. Retrieved May 30, 2016, from http://www.nursingworld.org/Mobile/Code-of-Ethics.

Bostan, S., Acuner, T., & Yilmaz, G. (2007). Patient (Customer) Expectations in Hospitals. *Health Policy, 82*(1), 62–70.

Burston, A. S., & Tuckett, A. G. (2013). Moral Distress in Nursing: Contributing Factors, Outcomes and Interventions. *Nursing Ethics, 20*(3), 312–324.

Creswell, J. W. (2007). *Qualitative Inquiry and Research Design: Choosing Among Five Approaches*. Thousand Oaks: Sage.

Daiski, I. (2004). Changing Nurses' Dis-empowering Relationship Patterns. *Journal of Advanced Nursing, 48*(1), 43–50.

De Raeve, L. (2002). Trust and Trustworthiness in Nurse-Patient Relationships. *Nursing Philosophy, 3*(2), 152–162.

Duttweiler, S. (2007). Vom Patienten zum Kunden? Ambivalenzen einer aktuellen Entwicklung. *Psychotherapeut, 52*(2), 121–126.

Hörnsten, A., Sandström, H., & Lundman, B. (2004). Personal Understandings of Illness Among People with Type 2 Diabetes. *Journal of Advanced Nursing, 47*(2), 174–182.

Ingadottir, B. (2009). *Adherence in Diabetes: Challenges, Negotiations and Dialogues. A Phenomenological Study on the Concept of Adherence from Patients' Perspective*. Saarbrücken: Lambert Academic Publishing.

Kälvemark, S., Höglund, A. T., Hansson, M. G., Westerholm, P., & Arnetz, B. (2004). Living with Conflicts-Ethical Dilemmas and Moral Distress in the Health Care System. *Social Science & Medicine, 58*(6), 1075–1084.

Kramer, M., & Schmalenberg, C. (2003). Securing "Good" Nurse/Physician Relationships. *Nursing Management, 34*(7), 34–38.

Maio, G. (2009). Dienst am Menschen oder Kunden-Dienst? Ethische Grundreflexionen zur sich wandelnden ärztlichen Identität. In C. Katzenmeier & K. Bergoldt (Eds.), *Das Bild des Arztes im 21. Jahrhundert* (pp. 21–35). Berlin: Springer.

Malloy, D. C., Hadjistavropoulos, T., McCarthy, E. F., Evans, R. J., Zakus, D. H., Park, I., Lee, Y., & Williams, J. (2009). Culture and Organizational Climate: Nurses' Insights into Their Relationship with Physicians. *Nursing Ethics, 16*(6), 719–733.

McDonald, J., Jayasuriya, R., & Harris, M. F. (2012). The Influence of Power Dynamics and Trust on Multidisciplinary Collaboration: A Qualitative Case Study of Type 2 Diabetes Mellitus. *BMC Health Service Research.* Retrieved May 30, 2016, from http://www.biomedcentral.com/1472-6963/12/63.

Miles, M. B., Huberman, A. M., & Saldana, J. (2013). Within-Case Displays: Exploring and Describing. In M. B. Miles, A. M. Huberman, & J. Saldana (Eds.), *Qualitative Data Analysis: An Expanded Sourcebook* (pp. 90–142). Thousand Oaks: Sage.

Mol, A. (2008). *The Logic of Care: Health and the Problem of Patient Choice.* New York: Routledge.

Moser, A., van der Bruggen, H., & Widdershoven, G. (2006). Competency in Shaping One's Life: Autonomy of People with Type 2 Diabetes Mellitus in a Nurse-Led, Shared-Care Setting: A Qualitative Study. *International Journal of Nursing Study, 43*(4), 417–427.

Okello, D. R., & Gilson, L. (2015). Exploring the Influence of Trust Relationships on Motivation in the Health Sector: A Systematic Review. *Human Resources for Health, 13*, 16–34.

Olshansky, E., Sacco, D., Fitzgerald, K., Zinkmund, S., Hess, R., Bryce, C., McTigue, K., & Fischer, G. (2008). Living with Diabetes. Normalizing the Process of Managing Diabetes. *The Diabetes Education, 34*(6), 1004–1012.

Parker, J. M. (1999). Patient or Customer: Caring Practices in Nursing and the Global Supermarket of Care. *Collegian, 6*(1), 16–23.

Pendry, P. S. (2007). Moral Distress: Recognizing It to Retain Nurses. *Nursing Economics, 25*(4), 217–221.

Pullon, S. (2008). Competence, Respect and Trust: Key Features of Successful Interprofessional Nurse-Doctor Relationships. *Journal of Interprofessional Care, 22*(2), 133–147.

Raspe, H. (1999). Patienten—Klienten—Kunden—Verbraucher. Sozialmedizinische Anmerkungen zu Beziehungsformen zwischen Kranken und Therapeuten. In A. Dörries (Ed.), *Patienten oder Kunden?* (pp. 9–19). Rehburg-Loccum: Evangelische Akademie Loccum.

Rich, K. (2008). Introduction to Bioethics, Nursing Ethics, and Ethical Decision-Making. In J. Butts & K. Rich (Eds.), *Nursing Ethics: Across the Curriculum and into Practice* (pp. 39–80). London: Jones & Bartlett Learning.

Robin, J. H., Callister, L. C., Berry, J. A., & Dearing, K. A. (2008). Patient-Centered Care and Adherence: Definitions and Applications to Improve Outcomes. *Journal of American Academic Nurse Practice, 20*(12), 600–607.

Rørtveit, K., Hansen, B. S., Leiknes, I., Joa, I., Testad, I., & Severinsson, E. (2015). Patients' Experiences of Trust in the Patient-Nurse Relationship—A Systematic Review of Qualitative Studies. *Open Journal of Nursing, 5*, 195–209.

Ryl, L., & Horch, K. (2013). Informiert und zufrieden?—Auf dem Weg zum mitbestimmenden Nutzer des Gesundheitswesens. *Umwelt und Menschen Informationsdienst, 2*, 111–117. Retrieved July 15, 2016, from http://edoc.rki.de/oa/articles/rel3ottiLPdA/PDF/26zIiui31EOuI.pdf.

Shigaki, C., Kruse, R. L., Mehr, D., Sheldon, K. M., Bin, G., Moore, C., & Lemaster, J. (2010). Motivation and Diabetes Self-Management. *Chronic Illness, 6*(3), 202–214.

Smith, A. S. (2012). Nurse Competence: A Concept Analysis. *International Journal of Nursing Knowledge, 23*(3), 172–182.

Thompson, I. E., Melia, K. M., Boyd, K. M., & Horsburgh, D. (2006). Power and Responsibility in Nursing Practice and Management. In I. E. Thompson (Ed.), *Nursing Ethics* (pp. 77–100). London: Churchill Livingstone.

Torpie, K. (2014). Customer Service vs. Patient Care. *Patient Experience Journal, 1*(2), 6–8.

Tronto, J. C. (2010). Creating Caring Institutions: Politics, Plurality, and Purpose. *Ethic and Social Welfare, 4*(2), 158–171.

Tscheulin, D. K., & Dietrich, M. (2010). Das Management von Kundenbeziehungen im Gesundheitswesen. In D. Georgi & K. Hadwich (Eds.), *Das Management von Kundenbeziehungen im Gesundheitswesen. Perspektiven—Analysen—Strategien—Instrumente* (pp. 253–276). Berlin: Springer.

Von Korff, M., Gruman, J., Schaefer, J., Curry, S. J., & Wagner, E. H. (1997). Collaborative Management of Chronic Illness. *Annals of Internal Medicine, 127*(12), 1097–1102.

Wagner, D., & Bear, M. (2009). Patient Satisfaction with Nursing Care: A Concept Analysis Within a Nursing Framework. *Journal of Advanced Nursing, 65*(3), 692–701.

Open Access This chapter is licensed under the terms of the Creative Commons Attribution 4.0 International License (http://creativecommons.org/licenses/by/4.0/), which permits use, sharing, adaptation, distribution and reproduction in any medium or format, as long as you give appropriate credit to the original author(s) and the source, provide a link to the Creative Commons license and indicate if changes were made.

The images or other third party material in this chapter are included in the chapter's Creative Commons license, unless indicated otherwise in a credit line to the material. If material is not included in the chapter's Creative Commons license and your intended use is not permitted by statutory regulation or exceeds the permitted use, you will need to obtain permission directly from the copyright holder.

Caring About Care in the Hospital Arena and Nurses' Voices in Hospital Ethics Committees: Three Decades of Experiences

Helen Kohlen

Introduction

Debates about care from an ethical perspective evolved in the 1980s and the work by Carol Gilligan (1982) and Nel Noddings (1984) in particular were influential in healthcare (Gallagher 2014; Kohlen 2009). In the USA at the same time, the inclusion of nurses in clinical ethics deliberations and their participation in Hospital Ethics Committees (HECs) was demanded so as to bring in their voice (Aroskar 1984; Fost and Cranford 1985; President's Commission 1983; Youngner et al. 1983).

Over the past 30 years, many countries have encouraged or mandated hospitals to have multi-professional HECs. For example, in Germany, the German Lutheran and Catholic Church Association published in 1997 a joint recommendation brochure to establish HECs (Deutscher Evangelischer Krankenhausverband and Katholischer Krankenhausverband 1997). Significant functions of HECs are to conduct ethics consultations, patient care review, develop policies and

H. Kohlen (✉)
Lehrstuhl Care Policy und Ethik, Philosophisch-Theologische Hochschule Vallendar (PTHV), Vallendar, Germany

© The Author(s) 2018

F. Krause, J. Boldt (eds.), *Care in Healthcare*,
https://doi.org/10.1007/978-3-319-61291-1_12

organize ethics education. The committees usually meet once a month at a certain time and place in the hospital.

Engagement in caring about care in the hospital arena from an ethical perspective and trying to bring in nurses' voices in HECs can be seen as a reaction to care deficits and loosening care practices that harm patients. Nurses in countries with distinctly different healthcare systems like Germany, Norway, the USA and Canada report similar shortcomings in their work environments and the quality of hospital care. A study in 2001 of more than 43,000 nurses practicing in more than 700 hospitals in 5 countries indicates that fundamental problems in the organization of work are widespread in hospitals in Europe and North America (Aiken et al. 2001, 2013). Maria Schubert and her colleagues (2008) as well as Beatrice Kalisch (2006) even refer to "missed nursing care".

Nurses reported spending time performing functions that did not call upon their professional training (delivering and retrieving food trays or transporting patients), while care practices requiring their skills and expertise (oral hygiene, skin care) were left undone (Aiken et al. 2001).

Studies in Canadian hospitals reveal what actually happens to nurses' care-giving in a hospital that is organized to be both efficient and effective in the use of its resources (Rankin and Campbell 2006). What emerges is a troubling picture for those who value and conceptualize care as a core practice for those who are dependent and vulnerable (Kittay 1999; Tronto 1993).

In this chapter, nurses' ethical problems in hospital care and their participation in HECs are traced over the last 30 years on the basis of studies in nursing ethics. HECs are seen as a discursive space to bring ethical problems to a head, including conflicts of care. Nurses' voices of care are illustrated using a field study in Germany (Kohlen 2009) as an example. While studies of nurses' participation in HECs can be traced back to the 1980s, investigations into their ethical concerns in hospital care go back to the 1990s.

Nurses' Ethical Concerns in Hospital Care

The dominant concerns found in stories and narratives of everyday nursing practice are of caring, responsiveness to others and responsibility (Benner et al. 1996). When the nurse ethicist and director of the Kennedy

Institute Carol Taylor (1997) interviewed nurses to get to know their ethical concerns, she had to realize that most of the nurses felt hard-pressed to describe the nature of their everyday nursing concerns that had ethical significance. She states that "...while some everyday nursing concerns are unique to nursing, most derive from tensions that involve the interdisciplinary team and raise broader issues about the human well-being that are best addressed by the institution or health care system at large" (Taylor 1997, p. 69). In order to investigate their concerns, she analysed collected case studies which lead nurses to request ethical consultation. She identified that nurses mostly struggle for the respect for human dignity, a commitment to holistic care, a commitment to individualized care which is responsive to unique needs of the patient, the responsibility for a continuity of care and the scope of authority and identifying the limits of care-giving (Taylor 1997, pp. 69–82). Taylor discusses that none of the concerns are unique to nursing, but they may be experienced with greater immediacy and urgency by nurses as well as other care-givers. She also observed that more nurses described their moral orientation as care-based rather than justice-based (see also Holly 1986).

Conflicts and Invisibilities

Both nurse ethicists Joan Liaschenko (1993) and Patricia Rodney (1997) have specifically investigated the concerns of practicing nurses. In an ethnographic study of nurses practicing on two acute medical units, Rodney explored the situational constraints that made it difficult for nurses to uphold their professional standards. Varcoe et al. (2004) support their findings of the serious structural and interpersonal constraints experienced, for example, excessive workloads for nurses, the absence of interdisciplinary team rounds, conflicts between team members inside and outside nursing and conflicts with patients and family members. Rodney (1997) explains that the inability of nurses to arrange space to talk with patients constrains their ability to truly focus and be attentive to the authentic needs of the patients and families. In a further study with her colleagues (Storch et al. 2002), in addition to a lack of time, another predominant theme was nurses' concern about appropriate use of resources. They struggled with decisions made by others regarding the allocation of scarce resources. Some of the nurses interviewed described physicians as not willing to listen to or to receive the nurses' point of view and were reluctant to accept that nurses have any independent moral responsibility when caring for patients (Storch et al. 2002). Moreover, the study gives evidence that the organizational climate, including policy development, is problematic for nurses. Sometimes this is related to a lack of policy, sometimes to the presence of a binding policy, and more often, to an ambiguous policy. For example, policies that were considered to be too binding, such as resuscitation policies, were related to patients whose best interest was overseen by following a code (Storch et al. 2002).

Central to the concerns given voice by nurses interviewed in Liaschenko's study was their sensitivity to patient need. They were aware of the

> … increased vulnerability to loss of … agency in the face of disease, illness. … Need was not seen solely in terms of a biomedical model of altered physiology but was conceived broadly to include those things which helped the individual to initiate or re-establish routines of lived experience and to cope with the settings in which they found themselves. … In this view, need was relative to the realities of the patient's day-to-day life. (Liaschenko 1993, p. 262)

Liaschenko (1993), Rodney (1997) and Varcoe et al. (2003) identified meeting the patients' and families' needs for emotional support as being undervalued and overlooked in nursing work. "Because emotional work is a social transaction and not a product, it is invisible in a product-driven society. New nurses learn very quickly what the 'official' work is and what the unofficial work is. Emotional work is extra, frequently coming out of the personal time of nurses" (Liaschenko 2001, p. 2). The authors argue that economically driven changes imply that only certain processes are remunerated. Consequently, only certain, measurable aspects of care are accounted for and funded, while other tasks of nursing care are ignored. Hereby, different values underlie what is accounted for and what is overlooked in an evaluation and a decision-making process that follows rather managerial rules (Rankin and Campbell 2006). Dealing with social issues that actually have no place in the sphere of medicine and the mandate of the hospital, like homelessness and poverty, is also invisible in nursing work (Varcoe et al. 2003).

Moral Distress, Missed Connectedness and Fragmentation of Care

According to several research findings, there are significant personal costs associated with nurses' caring work and concerns: fatigue, guilt and personal risk as well as the experience of anger, frustration and feelings of powerlessness (Erlen 1993; Redman 1996; Rodney 1997). Nurses feel frustrated because they cannot do what they should do with regard to "good care" and nurses feel powerless to affect their working conditions (Rodney 1997). The constraints limited the competences of nurses to care and resulted in moral distress, that is knowing "... the right things to do, but institutional constraints make it nearly impossible to pursue the right course of action" (Jameton 1984, p. 6). Moral distress is experienced by practitioners when they confront structural and interpersonal constraints in their workplaces (Aiken et al. 2000; Gaudine et al. 2011; Rodney and Varcoe 2001). Lorraine Hardingham (2004) argues that nurses often find themselves in positions where they have to compromise their moral integrity in order to survive in the hospital or other healthcare environment. The consequences are a fragmentation of care as well as fragmented decision-making that can have negative effects for patients and families and foster feelings of powerlessness and stress on the part of nurses (Varcoe et al. 2003). Nevertheless, institutional constraints cannot be interpreted as a justification for leaving out nursing caring practices, but can only be an explanation that needs further investigation.

In the study, *Power, Politics, and Practice: Towards a Better Moral Climate for Health Care Delivery*, Patricia Rodney (2005) identifies the main problems that prevent safe nursing practice. She emphasizes the dangerousness of "normalization":

> This means that serious congestion of patients in the ED, mismatches of patient acuity to available treatment / care, and overall lack of resources have started to become taken for granted. For instance, when asking hospital management for extra staff or to look for beds, nurses have told us (and we have seen) that the rebuttal is sometimes 'well, it was much worse the other day'. Nurses are sometimes asked to care for more than one ventilated patient plus other patients – a situation that would certainly not be considered 'normal' in a critical care unit. And patients are being held in

> the halls for so long now that some physicians are asking to start treatment in the hall or rapid treatment area without nursing coverage or assessment. This is in violation of safe emergency practice standards. Furthermore, it has become too much the norm that patients and their families will have to put up with far less than optimal care in our currently over-stretched provincial health care system. (Rodney 2005, p. 2)

Moreover, she points out that nurses describe themselves as being disconnected to their colleagues, management, other departments in the hospital or the community and that they feel that they have no meaningful say in how the emergency department is run, but are rather expected to put up with the consequences. Feeling connected and building up relationships in healthcare are important factors of healthcare outcomes for patients and the quality of work life experienced by healthcare providers (Varcoe et al. 2003, p. 959).

One reason is that nurses' issues of concern are systematic, that is to say: the problems arise in predictable settings and not randomly. The organization can make it very difficult for nurses to fulfil their ideals of good care. The ones who carry out caring work find it impossible to approach care as a coherent process. The fragmentation of care threatens the unity of the caring process. It is not something in the nature of *care-giving* itself, but rather the low social status and the poor organization of care that can make nursing a difficult practice. Are there practices of resistance?

Practices of healthcare providers can be resistant to imposed rules, changes and dominant ways of thinking. In these situations, for example, individual nurses ignored rules and the system in order to practice care according to the needs of patients and families. Canadian researchers give the example of emergency nurses' practices of "bending the rules" to give patients pain medication to take home despite the lack of a physicians' order (Varcoe et al. 2003, p. 967). The resistant practices identified are going against both the prevailing ideologies and colleagues following them.

According to these studies, the goals and rules of the institution can become the driving force behind any kind of actions and procedures whereby nurses act as facilitators and negotiators who are no longer dedicated to the well-being of patients, but to the system of management that implies a kind of control over patients as cases. What does it mean to know the case in comparison to knowing the patient and the person?

Knowing the Case Versus Knowing the Patient and the Person

Case histories and case records are part of a larger development of administrative technologies that can be called knowledge devices, used in professional administrative practices. Procedures for writing them are manufactured in ways that records are collected according to standards so that the individual is put into categories and interpretative schemata. The facts are abstracted from the actual events that happen at a certain place and time. Dorothy Smith remarks that they are

> typically embedded in and integral to forms of organization where the immediate and day-to-day contact with the people to be processed is at the front line and involves subordinates, whereas decisions about those people are made by persons in designated positions of responsibility who lack such on-going direct contact. (Smith 1990, p. 89)

Structuring the case story in such a way that meets this form, Smith explains, is articulated to an organization of power and position in which some have authority to contribute to the production of the textual realities and others do not. "Those who are the objects of case histories are normally distinctively deprived ... those who have direct knowledge of the patient's life outside the hospital or of her daily routines in the hospital are least privileged to speak and be heard" (Smith 1990, p. 91).

Institutionalized hospital practices operate as information-based and as patient case knowledge that is business-oriented to make healthcare organizations successful, and are not necessarily consistent with caring. Nurses learn to leave out experience-based domestic elements of care that would disrupt the authoritative plan to meet desired outcomes (Rankin and Campbell 2014). The nurses are attentive to the required workflow and try to smooth over things that might disrupt it. They focus on the technologically structured work and miss other aspects of nursing activities that are unaccounted for in the formal plans, directions, documentation and requirements. "Any effort or use of time and nursing attention that is outside the institutional version of care becomes extraneous" (Rankin and Campbell 2014, p. 168).

Based on the analysis of their empirical research data, Joan Liaschenko and Anastasia Fisher (1999) differentiate between types of knowledge: the case, the patient and the person. Case knowledge they consider as generalized biomedical knowledge of anatomy, physiology, pathology, as well as therapeutics (Liaschenko and Fisher 1999, pp. 33–35). Liaschenko (1997) claims that case knowledge is disembodied knowledge. One could know, for example, all necessary facts about cardiac disease without perceiving that disease as being embodied in a particular individual. The disease is understood as a deviation from the biological norm. Fisher and Liaschenko unfold the idea of case knowledge:

> This case, or biomedical, knowledge is the primary knowledge of the contemporary health care system in that it legitimises the practice of medicine which, in turn, controls knowledge. It also legitimises that aspect of nursing work that is concerned with monitoring disease processes and therapeutic responses. (Liaschenko and Fisher 1999, p. 33)

This case knowledge is the standard against which the specific features of an individual care receiver are measured. The shift from case knowledge to patient knowledge is made when the care-giver encounters the actual body of the care-receiver and, in doing so, knowledge transcends case knowledge and grows to patient knowledge. The care of the patient at the bedside requires knowledge of how the disease is manifest in this particular patient. It includes any unique features of anatomy and physiology in this patient, and how this patient responds to care and treatments. Patient knowledge also implies knowing how things get done for the individual within and between institutions as well as knowledge of other care providers who are involved. The complexity of patient knowledge is based on "... the fact that its content is no longer limited to generalized case knowledge and the expectancies for action which it generates. Rather, it consists of the nurse's interaction with a particular body, the responses of which will be compared to generalized case knowledge" (Liaschenko and Fisher 1999, p. 36).

In contrast to case and patient knowledge, person knowledge is defined as knowledge of the individual within his or her personal biography (Brody 2002). It implies knowing something about what the specific history means to the individual. Studies revealed that person knowledge was used when there was some conflict between courses of action desired by the individual and those desired by the therapeutic team (physician, physiotherapist, social worker etc.). Person knowledge is useful for nurses "to defend their arguments for an alternative management of disease trajectories and to justify their actions when those actions support an individual's agency, even though this can conflict with established biomedical or institutional courses of action" (Liaschenko and Fisher 1999, p. 39). In other terms, this differentiation could be understood as a confusion of means and purpose. While the case knowledge assumes certain features that make up a certain profile of a person that fits the use of certain procedures, diagnostic techniques and therapeutic possibilities, the person knowledge assumes an individual whose own biography and voice count to understand the case. Within the logic of the case knowledge, the individual can become a means to an end since you watch out for a profile that fits your available or prospective answers. Within the logic of the person knowledge, the individual is the purpose and transitional means, and answers have to be found in the process of getting to know the individual by listening to his or her own voice and unique history. The person knowledge takes caring time and "understanding" becomes decisive, while case knowledge saves time and understanding becomes unnecessary. The organization of care serves to separate the individual from the context in which interactions take place. To be taken away from that context means to become detached from the context of one's living. It becomes the organization's business. Individual histories can be rendered invisible or abstracted into a package of reports.

Besides being resistant and bending the rules, nurses could articulate the dilemmas of and in nursing care practices within the hospital arena and bring in patient as well as person knowledge. Hospital Ethics Committees can offer such a forum and space for nurses' voices. Joan Tronto (2010) convincingly describes in her article on how to *create caring institutions* that this can never happen without a "rhetorical space" (Code 1995) or a "moral space" (Walker 1993, 1998) or "a political space" (Tronto 2010) within which caring issues can be debated.

Thinking along the lines of John Dryzek's idea (2000) of fostering a discursive way of communication and deliberation, I am in favour of a discursive space. HECs can serve as a discursive space in the sense that an expansive kind of communication is supported that allows unruly and contentious voices from the margins. The characteristics are: (1) the presence of a hitherto scarcely represented group and their voices increase among the actors who are in a position of decision-making; (2) the implication of inequality and power relationships being bound to traditions is seen as a problem to be expounded when issues are raised and struggles for attention occur; (3) participation becomes real rather than symbolic (Dryzek 2000, p. vi; Kohlen 2009, p. 159).

Nurses' Membership, Voice and Participation in Hospital Ethics Committees

From their start, Hospital Ethics Committees (HECs) have recognized the importance of including individuals from different backgrounds as members. The legitimacy of the nurse's participation and their potential contribution as members of these committees has been acknowledged. Nursing as well as medical literature pays attention to the benefits of including nurses in ethics deliberations (Aroskar 1984; Aroskar et al. 2004; Fost and Cranford 1985; Fowler 1997; President's Commission 1983; Youngner et al. 1983). Nurses are supposed to add further dimensions to the decision-making process because they are usually in close proximity to their patients and spend more time at the bedside than any other member of the healthcare team. What are the experiences of nurses with regard to membership, participation and contributing their voice?

> Membership indicates who can speak, whose opinions are counted, and whose discounted. Membership may determine even which issues are seen as legitimate ethical concerns and which are not. ... So, to say that a hospital has an ethics committee tells us very little unless we know as well: who serves on the committee and under what authority. (Bosk and Frader 1998, p. 16)

In 1991, a study on *Physicians' Attitudes Toward Hospital Ethics Committees* found that merely 69% believed that nurses should be members in clinical committees and only 59% thought that they should have access (Finkenbine and Gramelspacher 1991), and when the number of Hospital Ethics Committees rose drastically, the American nurse ethicists Barba Edwards and Amy Haddad (1988) remarked that the specific and unique ethical concerns of nurses had also not been adequately addressed by these multidisciplinary committees. Their issues were not framed as ethical issues and therefore excluded. The nurse ethicist Dianne Bartels et al. (1994) who co-chaired a Hospital Ethics Committee in Minnesota in the 1980s is convinced: "I do not think hospital nurses have trouble speaking up, they just need a place to show up. (…) you need a place to convene, and then, once you are there, people don't have trouble … representing their issues". She also thinks that the co-chair model equalizes power, expands interaction on the committees and increases the comfort of nurses to be able to speak up. "Moreover, nurses need to learn the language (spoken by ethicists)" (Kohlen 2009, p. 150).

Cheryl Holly (1986) found that nurses are forced to function at conventional levels in the bureaucratic organization of the hospital. It was seen as a failure when they were not able to define concerns related to their practice in terms of rights and justice. Nurses who attempted to operate from a base of caring and responsibility were relegated to a conventional role. Betty Sichel (1992) examined procedures, deliberations, goals and functions of Hospital Ethics Committees and realized that a model of rights and justice is not appropriate to describe ethical questions with regard to caring practices.

A study on the participation and perception of nurses in HECs gives a detailed overview that reveals changes compared to previous findings (Oddi and Cassidy 1990). The study was conducted in two phases. In the first phase, they determined the number of acute care hospitals in a Midwestern state that have HECs and obtained the names of the nurses who serve as members of these committees. In the second phase, they contacted individual nurses to assess the extent of their formal involvement in ethical decision-making as well as their perception of the role of the ethics committee within their institutions. Of the 148 responses from hospitals, 45% said they have an ethics committee. All hospitals reported that nurses serve on those committees. The average number of nurses was said to be 2. Nurses were invited to participate in the study by anonymously completing a brief questionnaire about their perceptions "… of how the ethics committee is involved with selected aspects of practice" (Oddi and Cassidy 1990, p. 309). Members were predominantly female, hold a master's degree and served in administrative or management roles. The mean age was 42 years with a range of 25–65 years. The majority reported that they were either appointed or had volunteered to serve on the committee. They also indicated that they served on the committee from 1 to 7 years, with an average tenure of 2 years. Academic preparation, continuing education and self-directed learning were declared to be the main ways in which nurse members learn about ethics. Completion of an ethics course at either the graduate or the undergraduate level was reported by more than half of the respondents. Most of them indicated that they had attended continuing education programs, conferences or workshops on ethics. All respondents indicated that they contribute comments and ideas to the committee's discussions. Only a few indicated that they sometimes contribute, over 40% stated that they usually contribute and nearly half of them stated that they always contribute to the discussion. Only 1.4% indicated that their inputs were rarely sought (Oddi and Cassidi 1990).

The nurses interviewed in a study by Storch and Griener (1992) were generally positive regarding the perceived potential of a HEC, but only a few nurses were actually aware of the presence of the ethics committees (see also Pederson et al. 2009). For example, at one hospital, 20 nurses out of a total of 361 respondents were not aware of any ethics education being offered by the hospital. The study found that differences in ease of access to HECs by healthcare professionals were particularly pronounced between physicians and nurses. Physicians seemed to have greater access to the ethics committees and were perceived to have more support from them. In contrast, nurses did not perceive themselves as having direct access to the committees for consultation. They believed that access would be through their supervisor. Even though these gatekeepers posed no significant barrier, a few nurses interviewed stated that they would be too intimidated to go to the committee (Storch and Griener 1992, p. 23).

Cornelia Fleming (1997) found: "In institutions with established Hospital Ethics Committees, nurses are routinely included as members; however, the number of nurses able to participate at this level is small and not proportionally representative of nurses in clinical practice" (Fleming 1997, p. 7). A problem evolves: it is not bedside nurses as actors of caring practices who participate in HECs, but nursing managers. While nurses in management may bring a broader view, the perspective of staff nurses may be lost if they are not adequately represented. This is in fact a contradiction in the given role of nurses pointed out above, since nursing managers do not know patients by direct contact and have textual case knowledge, instead of a patient and person knowledge.

Although an occupation may have an adequate numerical representation, there could be differential participation in terms of communication exchange, as the study by Charlotte McDaniel (1998) reveals with regard to the nurses' communication exchange frequency as members in four sample HECs examined. Nurses proportionately represented the same or more membership numbers as physicians and the frequency of nurses' communication exchange was comparatively modest in proportion. The nurses had one of the smallest proportions of communication exchanges. Although most of the nurse members contributed communication exchanges to a topic, there were also nurses who did not participate at all. Nevertheless, nurses rated their participation effectiveness quite highly. Although nurses were moderately communicative on the committees, McDaniel suggests: "... nurses are engaged, active, and selectively participating in the committee deliberations. Nurses appear to be comfortable with a less overtly active, yet representative numerical membership on the committees" (McDaniel 1998, p. 50). Further exploration of the content of nurses' communication showed that they participate most in the discussions regarding patient care review and much less with regard to policy formation and education. McDaniel argues that nurses, representing the single largest group of healthcare personnel, need to be involved in the policies and decisions that surround and affect their administrative and clinical practice (McDaniel 1998, p. 48).

Sarah-Jane Dodd (2004) and her colleagues investigated the extent to which nurses engage with regard to "ethical activism" and "ethical assertiveness". Ethical activism they defined as "actions directed toward reforming institutional policies and procedures, as well as attitudes of physicians and other medical staff, to create favourable climate for (nurses') participation in ethical deliberations" (Dodd et al. 2004, p. 17). Ethical assertiveness is defined as "actions to enter or facilitate ethics deliberations in which nurses have not been included, whether through personal initiative, coaching patients, advocating patients' wishes to others, or ethical case finding" (Dodd et al. 2004, p. 17). The researchers contend that these two kinds of involvement are vitally important if nurses want to expand their ethical roles. The results indicated that nurses are more likely to employ ethical assertiveness and ethical activism in settings that are already receptive to nursing participation. The authors recommend that nurses

> need to try to change the hospital environment so that it promotes, rather than discourages, their participation. Even when not formally invited, (they) need to engage in ethical assertiveness when they advocate for patients, coach patients, act as ethical case finders, initiate ethics deliberations, and not withdraw from deliberations when not specifically asked to participate. (Dodd et al., 2004, p. 26)

The findings of the studies raise questions. First, why do the nurses know so little about ethics committees? Storch and Griener ask whether this goes back to a lack of knowledge that is induced by medical politics or whether it could be understood as a strategy of nursing administration maternalism that keeps staff nurses and head nurses removed from such information, or whether it might be simply a problem in communication within the hospital (Storch and Griener 1992, p. 25). In a study by Gaudine et al. (2011), nurses still report about a lack of knowledge about HECs as well as lack of experience.

A second question is whether ethics committees support existing structures and power relationships in the hospital rather than a shift to a democratic way of multi-professional discussion of ethical dilemmas and conflicts of care. The comments from physicians, nurses and administrators give credence to the view that HECs merely support the existing power structures.

The standards issued by the Joint Commission on Accreditation of Healthcare Organizations in 1992 required that structures be in place within institutions to enable nurses to participate in ethical deliberations (Erlen 1993). The standard is also included in the Standards of Clinical Nursing Practice developed by the American Nurses Association in 1991. But, having structures in place for nurses' participation does not necessarily mean that their voices are heard and that they bring in issues of care. The nurse ethicist and nursing manager Hans de Ruyter who has more than ten years of committee experiences in two different hospitals has gained a rather critical perspective and explains:

> Nurses' issues get addressed if they present them the way that the people, the physicians and the kind of the leadership see it. So, you have to present it in a certain way, and if you go outside of that model, ... so, if you bring up an issue that they do not classify as being an ethical issue, you don't get listened to. But people and nurses, I think, we are very adaptable, so there is [sic] always nurses that will learn the language and you get listened to (...) But then, you cannot truly bring up the issues that you think are ethical issues because it's very much I think with ethical issues which issues are classified as ethical issues and which ones aren't. And, I think that the nurses who do that and I can't talk about ...their mind, but for me, the quandary is, do I want to be a part of the leadership and then I have to adapt, or do I speak what I think should be spoken, and that automatically makes me an outsider. (Kohlen 2009, p. 155)

Nursing Ethics Committees

Some nursing professionals established Nursing Ethics Committees (NECs) as entities separate from the multi-professional HECs. These committees are structured within the healthcare organization created specifically to assist nurses in resolving ethical dilemmas. They are comprised of nurses who represent different positions of nurses within the organization, such as nurse managers, nurse educators as well as staff nurses. They are supposed to assist nurses to identify, clarify and articulate the issues in their practice (Erlen 1993; Fleming 1997).

A forerunner of this idea dates back to the time when the institutionalization of HECs after the Quinlan decision first subsided. At that time, in many hospitals, some still rather small and unknown groups began to meet regularly to discuss clinical problems they were facing with their colleagues (Kohlen 2009). The nurse ethicist Ruth Purtilo at Massachusetts General Hospital (MGH) in Boston looks back to the mid-1970s and explains:

> A group of nurses came to me telling 'We need an informal committee', … what they needed, was a room and time to talk about daily conflicts and dilemmas in clinical practice. We established an informal forum to discuss nursing ethical issues. The goal was to get this forum more or less institutionalized. One effect of the forum was the reduction of moral distress. (Kohlen 2009, p. 156)

One of the first official NECs was established in a Catholic hospital in Omaha, Nebraska in 1984. The vice president of patient care took the initiative to establish a NEC at the hospital, because she could not get the multi-professional ethics committee get moving (Kohlen 2009, p. 156). Amy Haddad, professor and director of the Center of Health Policy and Ethics at Creighton University in Omaha, and at that time doctoral student of nursing, became a consultant. She explains in an interview:

> … once the Nursing Ethics Committee was started and had a full day orientation to what ethics was, how decisions would be made, how to structure it (…) we had representatives from all the nursing areas in the hospital. This was before the hospital had governance structures, so there wasn't anything else in place (…) we got the people who were most interested to do it. So, we probably met for six months, people on board for (…) physicians to establish the institutional ethics committee. So, I had to work as a consultant to that committee (…) both committees, the nursing committee and the committee for the whole institution. (Kohlen 2009, p. 157)

NECs are described as a way to empower nurses so that they can more fully participate in multidisciplinary ethical discussions and prepare nurses to become effectively involved in HECs (Zink and Titus 1994, p. 70). On the basis of the descriptions, establishing NECs seems to be an adequate way to address ethical issues including the ones that refer to caring practices. But critical considerations are also expressed. Erlen argues that nurses who only discuss issues with other nurses might be limited in their focus. Perspectives given by other healthcare workers could challenge the analysis of the conflict and broaden the enquiry. "Although all nurses do not hold the same exact philosophy of nursing, there is a greater likelihood that there will be less divergence of perspectives and fewer alternatives presented when an ethics committee is comprised almost entirely of nurses" (Erlen 1997, p. 59). NECs might encourage division rather than collaboration with other disciplines (Fleming 1997, p. 8). The clinical ethicist, Mary Faith Marshall points out, that "nurses can be their best enemies, … a democratic process should be learnt … (and a) change in practices of local multi-disciplinary committees need to be supported by everyone" (Kohlen 2009, p. 157).

A closer look reveals that the question could be raised whether the functions of Nursing Ethics Committees are often the responsibility of other committees within the healthcare organizations. Moreover, while some nursing concerns are unique to nursing, most raise broader questions about human well-being that might be better addressed by the institution and the healthcare system at large (Taylor 1997, p. 69). A restricted discussion of these concerns to NECs may end up in their becoming trivialized or even marginalized. And, a separate nursing committee might communicate the image to the institution that these concerns are of lesser importance than those addressed by an interdisciplinary committee.

What happens if the committee actually serves to make nurses grow stronger in articulating their thoughts and put their issues of concern on the agenda? Haddad tells her piece of the story in an interview:

> It created problems over the years because they stood up, collectively, you know, so you got now five people on the unit, and they are not only five people, they are five experienced people because usually people that volunteer for this had been there a while. And now we are going through years of running the committee, and learning a language and all that. Then you got five people who were saying, we are not going to put up with this. They started to present problems (and there came a new director). She was

> unhappy with how they (the nurses) reacted to (…). I mean, they had learnt to ask questions. They had learnt to say that they would not agree on policies: We are not following it. Why are we not following it in this case, so what is happening? They had learnt to use tools of good arguments. (...) They had been taught to tell why (...) you cannot go up to somebody and say you are wrong, you have to have good arguments, and be able to say, here are my concerns and this is why (...) and they had been taught to do that, and they had learnt to link arms in how to do that, because nobody wants to be the one going forward. (Kohlen 2009, p. 158)

Bart Cusveller (2012) studied HECs and nurses' competency profiles. For future development, nurses ask for education in communication skills for all committee members, such as listening, speaking and writing. The ethics committee nurses were confronted with issues arising from constraints in the institutional context, such as budget issues and staff shortages.

In summary, the research findings about nurses' participation in HECs show that their participation does not necessarily mean that their issues are raised and their voices are heard. The following example taken from a field study in Germany (Kohlen 2009) can illustrate how caring issues are minimized and dismissed.

Voices of Care in a German Hospital Ethics Committee: A Petit Ethical Problem

A retrospective case consultation takes place in a committee meeting in a German hospital (Kohlen 2009, pp. 188–192):

A nurse had written down a concern in order to consult the committee. The female minister took the paper to the committee meeting and read it aloud. The nurse had experienced a situation two years ago that was still bothering her: An elderly female patient had been in need of a blood bottle. When the blood bottle arrived from the lab, it was still very cold, and the physician on shift asked the nurse to put the bottle on the old lady's belly, so that the blood bottle would warm up easily for her. The nurse, who did know the patient, could not imagine doing it. The patient had been sleeping and was not in an alert condition at all. The female physician then told her to ask another nurse to do it, someone who would be more professional than her.

The discussion in the ethics committee developed as followed:

Female Minister:	"It is really uncomfortable to have something cold on your belly!"
Physician A:	"This is absurd from a medical perspective. There are, of course, other technical aids that can help to warm up blood bottles".
Nurse A:	"This nurse feels like an advocate for the patient, and wants to take care of her autonomy".
Physician A:	"This is really a mini ethical problem!"
Physician B:	"I think the problem emerged from hierarchy!"
Minister A:	"I think they have some communication problems on the ward".
Physician C:	"But this is really a petit ethical problem!"

The discussion ends after some minutes, declaring that this is really a minor problem. The minister explains that she will have to talk to the nurse who has revealed her concern.

Female Minister asks:	"What should I tell her?
Physician A:	"You can tell her that she did not do anything wrong within the current knowledge of practice".
Physician B:	"And you can add that the problem had to do with hierarchy and failed communication".
Physician C adds:	"Well, the more I think about it, the more I feel instrumentalized by this nurse, because this is not an ethical problem at all!"
Nurse B:	"You can tell that she did not do anything wrong, and you can tell her about the possible hierarchy and communication problem behind it, but never tell her that this is not or is just a small ethical problem".

The meeting abruptly ends; people rose from their places and left the room. The minister remained there and took some notes.

Interpretation

First, the minister reacts and states, "It is really uncomfortable to have something cold on your belly". And this actually collides with a practice of care that does not allow one to put somebody into an uncomfortable state for the use of something or somebody else. The lady who is ill and sleeping cannot defend herself and therefore needs protection. The physician explicitly speaks from a medical perspective, stating that "this is absurd" and that this is not the right way to warm up blood bottles, because there are technical aids. He clarifies that this is obviously not a medical dilemma in which physicians do not know how to make an adequate decision.

Nurse A shows empathy for the nurse who has revealed her concern. She identifies the role of the nurse who cared for the old lady as an "advocate for the patient" who wanted to take care of her autonomy. Caring for her autonomy from a nursing understanding could mean that the patient cannot articulate herself and therefore needs protection, here given by the nurse. This is a mandate of nurses. It is different from the physician's, who is interested in getting a warm blood bottle for a medical intervention. Nursing care for patients who are sleeping implies keeping her or him in a state as comfortable as possible while protecting them from disturbing noises, interventions that can be postponed like "taking the blood pressure", as well as disturbing and uncomfortable interventions like putting a cold blood bottle on their warm belly. Although, in the patient's current state of not being able to verbally interact, the nurse sees that her autonomy still belongs to her and cannot be taken away, she uses the principle of autonomy to justify her nursing care, namely, her responsibility to take care of the patient's sleep.

When the physician defines the situation as "a mini ethical problem" without giving any reason, no questions or controversial points are raised. Why this is only a small ethical problem is left open. The physician does not feel a need for explanation, and nobody else asks for it. Then the commentaries that lack explanation move on: Physician B declares it as a problem that has to do with hierarchy, and Minister A remarks that the problem might be linked to "some communication problems on the ward". Since the exclamations that follow the non-rejected definition of a "mini ethical problem", one could ask whether hierarchy and communication are categories that can be put under the umbrella of small ethical problems or whether they are indicators for difficult situations that cannot simply be framed as ethical. Framing them in the context of small ethical problems minimizes their potential for conflicts and understanding the situation in its complexity which, of course, can harm not only patients but also disrupt professional identities, here nursing care.

When Physician C repeats the remark of Physician A that this is a "petit ethical problem", the conversation is closed down. There seems to be a hidden consensus about how much time should be spent on what kind of issues. That the discussion of the concern does not deserve much time could have been evoked by the minimization of the problem. The minister, realizing that the discussion is ending, asks the rather pragmatic question: "What should I tell her?" and the first answer is given by Physician A who started to comment on the concern. "You can tell her that she did not do anything wrong...", he authorizes the minister to tell. Does this mean that the nurse acted correctly according to a medical perspective? What are the criteria to distinguish between wrong and right in this situation? And who has the power to define it?

Physician B adds that the nurse should be told that "the problem had to do with hierarchy and failed communication". What is the message of this information? What can the nurse take out of this kind of analysis? This is difficult to tell, because there is no explanation. With regard to inter-relationships, especially between different professions, you can narrow down and contextualize nearly everything with hierarchy and communication problems in a hospital. Physician C "feels instrumentalized" by the concern of the nurse. This is a strong reproach. "This is not an ethical problem at all!" is the explanation for his feeling. Does a talk of problems which are not defined as ethical ones, instrumentalize disputants? Again, it is not clear what counts as a "real ethical problem" in comparison to a "petit" ethical problem, or a different kind of a problem, for example, of competence and communication. Criteria are not given. What is the legitimization to minimize the nursing concern at all?

It is the physician who has the power to declare what counts as a "real ethical problem" and what counts as a petit ethical problem. Nobody in the group asked for an explanation why the problem is declared to be a petit ethical problem. Nobody talks about the physician who told the nurse to use the warmth of a patient's body to warm up a blood bottle. What is her part in the story? What can be said about her clinical expertise and responsibility? Did she behave in a correct manner? Did she possibly think that this might be a "petit ethical problem" that counts less than the outcome, respectively, having a warm blood bottle for another patient in need?

The nurses' professional role is to take care of the patient's sleep. The nurse theorist Nancy Roper has developed a conceptual framework for nursing practice. One component of the model is called the "Activities of Daily Life" (ADL). Relaxing and being able to sleep is one element of these daily activities nurses have to care for. This involves having an eye on the duration of sleep, times of sleep, day and night rhythm, sleeping quality, rituals of falling asleep, habits and aids to fall asleep. Knowing the patient involves knowing his or her sleeping habits and knowing what this special patient needs to get the kind and duration of sleep that helps her to recover and gives comfort to her, especially when she is in pain and dying. The more dependent the patient is due to his situation of illness or disease, the more *comfort* the patient needs. For nurses, comfort implies a moral stance, clinical knowledge and the tangible, practical skills in which they have developed expertise.

Conclusion

The experiences of three decades caring about care in the hospital arena from an ethical perspective and trying to bring in nurses' voices into the discursive space of HECs point to structural shortcomings (resources), attention needing to be paid to power relationships and to the use of the ethical language being bound to a traditional institutional hierarchy in hospitals. Are structural shortcomings and the power-relationships expounded a problem in the first place? Is the language of ethics reflected to see whether issues of care can be described in depth? What are the theories and frameworks of ethics that rule the committee debates and how can they be broadened to capture issues of care?

Although the findings of my field study in Germany that investigated nurses' participation in HECs as illustrated above cannot be generalized, they support the assumption that ethical conflicts of delivering caring practices are not listened to as such. As a result, when framing a conflict of care as an ethical one, it is framed as a "petit ethical problem" and its importance for attention and consideration is therefore minimized.

Writing and talking about care mean that we need to take care of our care language and adapt it. It is difficult dealing with the limits of using words that do not represent patient knowledge, but only case knowledge that is textual and disembodied. Therefore, nurses who do bedside nursing and face-to-face body care need to be taken seriously whenever they articulate a concern about care.

References

Aiken, L. H., Clarke, S. P., & Sloane, D. M. (2000). Hospital Restructuring: Does It Adversely Affect Care and Outcomes? *Journal of Nursing Administration, 30*(10), 457–465.

Aiken, L. H., Clarke, S. P., Sloane, D. M., Sochalski, J. A., Busse, R., Clarke, H., Giovannetti, P., Hunt, J., Rafferty, A. M., & Shamian, J. (2001). Nurses' Reports on Hospital Care in Five Countries. *Health Affairs, 20*(3), 43–53.

Aiken, L. H., Sloane, D. M., Bruyneel, L., Van den Heede, K., & Sermeus, W. (2013). Nurses' Reports of Working Conditions and Hospital Quality of Care in 12 Countries in Europe. *International Journal of Nursing Studies, 50*(2), 143–153.

Aroskar, M. A. (1984). Health Care Professionals and Ethical Relationships on IECs. In R. E. Cranford & A. E. Doudera (Eds.), *Institutional Ethics Committees and Health Care Decision Making* (pp. 218–225). Michigan: Health Administration Press.

Aroskar, M. A., Moldow, G. D., & Good, C. M. (2004). Nurses' Voices: Policy, Practice and Ethics. *Nursing Ethics, 11*(3), 268–276.

Bartels, D., Youngner, S., & Levine, J. (1994). HealthCare Ethics Forum '94: Ethics Committees: Living Up to Your Potential. *AACN Clinical Issues in Critical Care Nursing, 5*(3), 313–323.

Benner, P. E., Tanner, C. A., & Chesla, C. A. (1996). *Expertise in Nursing Practice: Caring, Clinical Judgement, and Ethics*. New York: Springer.

Bosk, C., & Frader, J. (1998). Institutional Ethics Committees: Sociological Oxymoron, Empirical Black Box. In R. G. De Vries & J. Subedi (Eds.), *Bioethics and Society. Constructing the Ethical Enterprise* (pp. 94–116). New Jersey: Prentice Hall.

Brody, H. (2002). Narrative Ethics and Institutional Impact. In R. Charon & M. Montello (Eds.), *Stories Matter. The Role of Narrative in Medical Ethics* (pp. 149–153). New York: Routledge.

Code, L. (1995). *Rhetorical Spaces: Essays on Gendered Locations*. New York: Routledge.

Cusveller, B. (2012). Nurses Serving on Clinical Ethics Committees: A Qualitative Exploration of a Competency Profile. *Nursing Ethics, 19*(3), 431–442.

Deutscher Evangelischer Krankenhausverband e.V., & Katholischer Krankenhausverband Deutschlands e.V. (1997). *Ethik-Komitee im Krankenhaus*. Freiburg.

Dodd, S.-J., Jansson, B. S., Brown-Saltzman, K., Shirk, M., & Wunch, K. (2004). Expanding Nurses' Participation in Ethics: An Empirical Examination of Ethical Activism and Ethical Assertiveness. *Nursing Ethics, 11*(1), 15–27.

Dryzek, J. S. (2000). *Deliberative Democracy and Beyond. Liberals, Critics, Contestations*. Oxford: Oxford University Press.

Edwards, B. J., & Haddad, A. M. (1988). Establishing a Nursing Bioethics Committee. *Journal of Nursing Administration, 18*(3), 30–33.

Erlen, J. A. (1993). Empowering Nurses Through Nursing Ethics Committees. *Orthopaedic Nursing, 12*(2), 69–72.

Erlen, J. A. (1997). Are Nursing Ethics Committees Necessary? *HEC Forum, 9*(1), 55–67.

Finkenbine, R., & Gramelspacher, G. (1991). Physicians' Attitudes Toward Hospital Ethics Committees. *Indiana Medicine, 84*(11), 804–807.

Fleming, C. M. (1997). The Establishment and Development of Nursing Ethics Committees. *HEC Forum, 9*(1), 7–19.

Fost, N., & Cranford, R. E. (1985). Hospital Ethics Committees: Administrative Aspects. *Journal of the American Medical Association, 253*(18), 2687–2692.

Fowler, M. (1997). Nursing's Ethics. In A. J. Davis, M. A. Aroskar, J. A. Liaschenko, & T. S. Drought (Eds.), *Ethical Dilemmas and Nursing Practice* (pp. 17–34). New Jersey: Prentice Hall.

Gallagher, A. (2014). Moral Boundaries and Nursing Ethics. In G. Olthuis, H. Kohlen, J. Heier, & J. C. Tronto (Eds.), *Moral Boundaries Redrawn. The Significance of Joan Tronto's Argument for Political Theory, Professional Ethics, and Care as Practice* (pp. 133–149). Leuven: Peeters.

Gaudine, A., LeFort, S. M., Lamb, M., & Thorne, L. (2011). Ethical Conflicts with Hospitals: The Perspective of Nurses and Physicians. *Nursing Ethics, 18*(6), 756–766.

Gaudine, A., Lamb, M., LeFort, S. M., & Thorne, L. (2011). Barriers and Facilitators to Consulting Hospital Clinical Ethics Committees. *Nursing Ethics, 18*(6), 767–780.

Gilligan, C. (1982). *In a Different Voice. Psychological Theory and Women's Development*. Cambridge: Harvard University Press.

Hardingham, L. B. (2004). Integrity and Moral Residue: Nurses as Participants in a Moral Community. *Nursing Philosophy, 5*(2), 127–134.

Holly, C. M. (1986). *Staff Nurses' Participation in Ethical Decision Making: A Descriptive Study of Selected Situational Variables*. Ann Arbor: University Microfilms International.

Jameton, A. (1984). *Nursing Practice. The Ethical Issues*. New Jersey: Prentice Hall.

Kalisch, B. J. (2006). Missed Nursing Care: A Qualitative Study. *Journal of Nursing Care Quality, 21*(4), 306–313.

Kittay, E. F. (1999). *Love's Labor: Essays on Women, Equality and Dependency*. New York: Routledge.

Kohlen, H. (2009). *Conflicts of Care. Hospital Ethics Committees in the USA and Germany*. Frankfurt am Main: Campus.

Liaschenko, J. (1993). *Faithful to the Good: Morality and Philosophy in Nursing Practice*. Unpublished doctoral dissertation, University of California, San Francisco.

Liaschenko, J. (1997). Knowing the Patient? In S. Thorne & V. Hayes (Eds.), *Nursing Praxis. Knowledge and Action* (pp. 23–38). Thousand Oaks: Sage Publications.

Liaschenko, J. (2001). Thoughts on Nursing Work. *Bioethics Examiner, 5*(2), 2–6.

Liaschenko, J., & Fisher, A. (1999). Theorizing the Knowledge that Nurses Use in the Conduct of Their Work. *Scholarly Inquiry for Nursing Practice, 13*(1), 29–41.

McDaniel, C. (1998). Hospital Ethics Committees and Nurses' Participation. *Journal of Nursing Administration, 28*(9), 47–51.

Noddings, N. (1984). *Caring. A Feminine Approach to Ethics and Moral Education*. Berkeley: University of California Press.

Oddi, L. F., & Cassidy, V. R. (1990). Participation and Perception of Nurse Members in the Hospital Ethics Committee. *Western Journal of Nursing Research, 12*(3), 307–317.

Pederson, R., Akre, V., & Førde, R. (2009). Barriers and Challenges in Clinical Ethics Consultations: The Experiences of Nine Clinical Ethics Committees. *Bioethics, 23*(8), 460–469.

President's Commission for the Study of Ethical Problems in Medicine and Biomedical and Behavioural Research. (1983). *Deciding to Forego Life-Sustaining Treatment*. Washington DC: U.S. Government Printing Office.

Rankin, J., & Campbell, M. (2006). *Managing to Nurse: Inside Canada's Healthcare Reform*. Toronto: University of Toronto Press.

Rankin, J., & Campbell, M. (2014). Care and Gender in Nurses' Institutionally Organized Work. In G. Olthuis, H. Kohlen, J. Heier, & J. C. Tronto (Eds.), *Moral Boundaries Redrawn. The Significance of Joan Tronto's Argument for Political Theory, Professional Ethics, and Care as Practice* (pp. 153–173). Leuven: Peters.

Redman, B. K. (1996). Responsibility of Healthcare Ethics Committees Towards Nurses. *HEC Forum, 8*(1), 52–60.

Rodney, P. A. (1997). *Towards Connectedness and Trust: Nurses' Enactment of Their Moral Agency Within an Organizational Context*. Unpublished doctoral dissertation, University of British Columbia, Vancouver.

Rodney, P. (2005, September 6–8). *Power, Politics, and Practice: Towards a Better Moral Climate for Health Care Delivery*. The 9th International Philosophy of Nursing Conference, Book of Abstracts, University of Leeds.

Rodney, P., & Varcoe, C. (2001). Towards Ethical Inquiry in the Economic Evaluation of Nursing Practice. *Canadian Journal of Nursing Research, 33*(1), 35–57.

Schubert, M., Glass, T. R., Clarke, S. P., Schaffert-Witvliet, B., Sloane, D. M., & De Geest, S. (2008). Rationing of Nursing Care and Its Relationship to Patient Outcomes: The Swiss Extension of the International Hospital Outcomes Study. *International Journal for Quality in Health Care, 20*(4), 227–237.

Sichel, B. A. (1992). Ethics of Caring and the Institutional Ethics Committee. In H. Bequaert Holmes & L. M. Purdy (Eds.), *Feminist Perspectives in Medical Ethics* (pp. 113–123). Bloomington: Indiana University Press.

Smith, D. E. (1990). *The Conceptual Practices of Power. A Feminist Sociology of Knowledge*. Boston: Northeastern University Press.

Storch, J. L., & Griener, G. G. (1992). Ethics Committees in Canadian Hospitals: Report of the 1990 Pilot Study. *Healthcare Management Forum, 5*(1), 19–26.

Storch, J. L., Rodney, P., Pauly, B., Brown, H., & Starzomsky, R. (2002). Listening to Nurses' Moral Voices: Building a Quality Health Care Environment. *Nursing Leadership, 15*(4), 7–16.

Taylor, C. R. (1997). Everyday Nursing Concerns: Unique? Trivial? Or Essential to Healthcare Ethics? *HEC Forum, 9*(1), 68–84.

Tronto, J. C. (1993). *Moral Boundaries: A Political Argument for an Ethic of Care*. New York: Routledge.

Tronto, J. C. (2010). Creating Caring Institutions: Politics, Plurality, and Purpose. *Ethics and Social Welfare, 4*(2), 158–171.

Varcoe, C., Rodney, P., & McCormick, J. (2003). Health Care Relationships in Context: An Analysis of Three Ethnographies. *Qualitative Health Research, 13*(7), 957–973.

Varcoe, C., Doane, G., Pauly, B., Rodney, P., Storch, J. L., Mahoney, K., McPherson, G., Brown, H., & Starzomski, R. (2004). Ethical Practice in Nursing: Working the In-betweens. *Journal of Advanced Nursing, 45*(3), 316–325.

Walker, M. U. (1993). Keeping Moral Space Open: New Images of Ethics Consulting. *Hastings Center Report, 23*(2), 33–40.

Walker, M. U. (1998). *Moral Understandings. A Feminist Study in Ethics*. New York: Routledge.

Youngner, S. J., Jackson, D. L., Coulton, C., Juknialis, B. W., & Smith, E. (1983). A National Survey of Hospital Ethics Committees. In President's Commission for the Study of Ethical Problems in Medicine and Biomedical and Behavioural Research. In *Deciding to Forego Life-Sustaining Treatment* (pp. 443–449). Washington, DC: U.S. Government Printing Office.

Zink, M. R., & Titus, L. (1994). Nursing Ethics Committees—Where Are They? *Nursing Management, 25*(6), 70–76.

Open Access This chapter is licensed under the terms of the Creative Commons Attribution 4.0 International License (http://creativecommons.org/licenses/by/4.0/), which permits use, sharing, adaptation, distribution and reproduction in any medium or format, as long as you give appropriate credit to the original author(s) and the source, provide a link to the Creative Commons license and indicate if changes were made.

The images or other third party material in this chapter are included in the chapter's Creative Commons license, unless indicated otherwise in a credit line to the material. If material is not included in the chapter's Creative Commons license and your intended use is not permitted by statutory regulation or exceeds the permitted use, you will need to obtain permission directly from the copyright holder.

Towards a Three-Dimensional Perspective of Space for Humanizing Hospital Care

Hanneke van der Meide

Introduction

> The patient in the bed has almost become an icon for the real patient who is in the computer. I've actually coined a term for that entity in the computer. I call it the iPatient. The iPatient is getting wonderful care all across America. The real patient often wonders, where is everyone? When are they going to come by and explain things to me? Who's in charge? Everybody who enters the healthcare system becomes isolated—it is built into the very infrastructure of the system. And, following from this, we can see that one of the most helpful things we can do to improve the experience of bodily impairment is to reduce that social isolation and vulnerability.

This apt description voiced by the medical doctor Abraham Verghese in a TED Talk expresses a feeling that is palpable in wider society (Verghese 2011). Various scholars have described the alienating effect provoked by being in the hospital or in other care settings. A patient's sense of human belonging is likely to become vulnerable in an institu-

H. van der Meide (✉)
University of Humanistic Studies, Utrecht, The Netherlands

© The Author(s) 2018
F. Krause, J. Boldt (eds.), *Care in Healthcare*,
https://doi.org/10.1007/978-3-319-61291-1_13

tional context such as a hospital (Williams and Irurita 2004). This comes on top of the already disconcerting effect of the disease itself (Alzhén 2011; Svenaeus 2011). Illness has essentially been characterized as an experience of not feeling at home in the world or in one's body (Toombs 2001a). Sveneaus describes the body as uncanny. He draws upon Heidegger's description of illness as unhomelike being-in-the-world, but adds that the body will always remain *our* body. "The body is alien, yet, at the same time, myself. Although it involves biological processes beyond my control, these processes still belong to me as lived by me" (Svenaeus 2000). In this context, some authors state that features of contemporary healthcare might add extra suffering and leave patients with feelings of discomfort and even pain (Berglund et al. 2012; van Heijst 2011). Suffering can be distinguished from physical pain in that in physical pain, there can still be a sense of meaning and wholeness, while in suffering, people feel disconnected from others and the self (Cassell 2001).

Humanization refers to practices that take the perspectives and values of people who are part of the practice into consideration (Visse 2012). In this chapter I will limit myself to the notion of space and its meaning for the humanization of care. The influence of spatial aspects on patients' well-being is described as crucial for more humanizing care (Galvin and Todres 2013; Norlyk et al. 2013). The notion of lived space is usually introduced referring to "the more" of the physical space: the felt and experiential space (Norlyk et al. 2013). In Europe, over the last decade, a lifeworld awareness has increasingly been applied to healthcare. Care given from a lifeworld perspective could provide important ideas and values that are central to the humanization of healthcare practice. This lifeworld perspective is grounded in phenomenological philosophy, which I will briefly describe in this chapter, followed by an examination of how lived space is understood and illustrated by examples from empirical research. Second, from a care ethical perspective, I will argue for a broader notion of space that better reflects the practice of care. The lifeworld approach remains focused on care as too narrow an interaction between two people, the patient and the healthcare professional. Third, I will explore the three-dimensional perspective of space as described by philosopher and sociologist Henri Lefebvre. His view allows a shift in focus from the experiencing subject to social practice and changes the object of analysis when studying the (de)humanization of care.

Phenomenology and Lived Space

Lifeworld

Phenomenology refers to a philosophical attitude towards the world. "Phenomenology is the study of human experience and of the way things present themselves to us in and through such experience" (Sokolowski 2000). In contrast to Western scientific thinking, phenomenology aims to bring together polarities such as mind-body, subject-object, individual-social and feelings-thoughts. The hyphens signify intertwining rather than separation (Finlay 2011). This is why Merleau-Ponty describes phenomenology as a science of ambiguity. There is always ambiguity and, in a sense, indeterminacy, "precisely because we are not capable of disembodied reflection upon our activities, but are involved in an intentional arc that absorbs both our body and our mind" (Merleau-Ponty 1962). Heidegger describes the impossibility of being disconnected from the world by his concept of being-in-the-world. The lifeworld—*Lebenswelt*—is the central phenomenological focus and portrays this lived wholeness and inseparability. It denotes a meaningful whole that is both shared and experienced by individuals from their own unique perspective (Heidegger 1998).

The issue of the lifeworld should be understood against the background of the advent of modern science; before then, people simply thought that the world we live in was the only world there was (Sokolowski 2000). The project of phenomenology as started with Edmund Husserl (1859–1938) was to show that the exact, mathematical sciences are founded on the lifeworld and that they are transformations of the experience people directly have of things in the world. Husserl attempted to call to mind that

> the lifeworld (...) is always already there, existing in advance for us, the 'ground' of all praxis whether theoretical or extra theoretical. The world is

> pre-given to us (…) not occasionally but always and necessarily as the universal field of all actual and possible praxis, a lifeworld. To live is always to live-in-certainty-of-the word. (Husserl 1970, p. 142)

The lifeworld is the beginning place-flow from which we divide up our experiences into more abstract categories and names (Galvin and Todres 2013). Husserl did not question the value of modern science and his work suggests that there is nothing wrong with concepts and scientific theories as long as they refer to specific experiences and not just to each other. *Phenomenology* as a research method is directed towards exploring a human experience (a phenomenon) as it is lived through rather than how we conceptualize, theorize or reflect on it.

In recent years, interest in phenomenology has increased in the domain of professional practice (van Manen 2014). While in research primacy is increasingly given to categories, numbers and averages that might obscure the human dimensions (Galvin and Todres 2013), phenomenology can offer "a bridge across the chasm between practice and research" (Finlay 2011). Although not everyone explicitly refers to the phenomenological notion of lifeworld, Dahlberg, Todres and Galvin have done so. These Swedish and British researchers have revisited Husserl's notion of lifeworld and describe in various papers how care led from this perspective could provide important ideas and values that are central to the humanization of healthcare practice. Humanization refers to "those things which make us feel more human" (Galvin and Todres 2013). They define eight philosophically informed dimensions for the humanization of care: insiderness, agency, uniqueness, togetherness, sense-making, sense of personal journey, sense of place and embodiment. The corresponding dimensions of dehumanization are described as: objectification, passivity, homogenization, isolation, loss of meaning, loss of personal journey, sense of dislocation and a reductionist view of the body (Todres et al. 2009). They advocate a perspective of care what they call lifeworld-led care that should be distinguished from patient-led or person-centred healthcare (Dahlberg et al. 2009). Although they appreciate these perspectives that emphasize the agency of patients, they question whether they encompass the kinds of concerns and knowledge of patients. On the one hand, they argue a consumerist and citizen model overly emphasizes personal or collective agency and self-authority and underemphasizes patients as "exposed" and "vulnerable." In this way, they are an opposite reductionist version of a medical model that overemphasizes illness and underemphasizes the phenomenon of human agency. They contend that when people become patients, they want to be seen in both their agency and vulnerability and feel unmet by interactions that emphasize one or the other. Because of the space for ambiguity, a phenomenological lifeworld perspective can address both dimensions of human existence.

Lived Space as an Existential of the Lifeworld

The lifeworld is something both general and individual as we live in a shared world that we experience from our own unique perspective (van Manen 2014). To understand is both to understand something of this unique individual and the shared intersubjective horizons within which any unique experience occurs (Galvin and Todres 2013). Heidegger differentiates between the ontological that refers to the existential preconditions of being human and the ontic, in which there are many uniquely different individual and cultural ways of experiencing such ontological structures. Phenomenological research aims to give snapshots of these ontological structures, acknowledging that they always remain a part of the whole (Hansen 2015). There are at least four ontological structures described by various phenomenological philosophers that pervade the lifeworlds of all human beings, regardless of their historical, cultural or social situatedness. In order to not confuse these fundamental lifeworld themes with the more particular themes (*the ontic*) of certain human phenomena that are studied in phenomenological research, van Manen describes the fundamental lifeworld themes as "existentials" (van Manen 2014). Ashworth and Ashworth call them fragments to emphasize their interlinking, interpenetrating meanings (Ashworth and Ashworth 2003). Todres et al. use the words "constituents" and "dimensions" (Todres et al. 2007). They all refer to a conceptual framework that can be used in research to describe human experiences in their holistic context. The constituents of the lifeworld most commonly identified are lived time, lived space, lived body and lived intersubjectivity. These four existentials are proven to be a helpful guide for reflection in the research process of phenomenological questioning, reflecting and writing (van Manen 2014).

Lived space is thus considered an existential dimension of our lifeworld. Unlike objective space, which refers to dimensions such as length, height and depth, lived space refers to the perceptual experience of space. This lived space is difficult to put into words and yet we know that the space in which we find ourselves affects the way we feel. The huge space of, for example, a train station may make us feel exposed and small, and a nice and cosy restaurant lets us feel at ease. The typical (sterile) air we smell when we enter the hospital can reassure us or instil fear. What this lived space as felt space entails can best be illustrated by examples from research practice.

Example 1: Lived Space for a Person with Alzheimer
Ashworth and Ashworth describe the lifeworld of a person suffering from Alzheimer's disease in an attempt to focus in a realistic way on what people with dementia have rather than what they lack (Ashworth and Ashworth 2003). In order to care well for a person with dementia, a carer should become an informal phenomenologist and set aside his or her own criteria of truth and reality and suspend the scholarly knowledge of what dementia typifies. Instead, the carer turns his or her attention to the actual activity and talk of the person in order to discover the meanings of that person's lifeworld. They describe how, for a woman with dementia, space no longer radiates around her as the known and familiar or the available-to-be-known. Some spaces may be experienced as boundariless. There are, for example, no constraints of modesty or privacy. The woman in the study is no longer able to rely on space, and a gate or locked doors, for example, do not mean a boundary or threshold. "Naming a space may no longer have the power to reassure – the label may no longer indicate 'here' versus 'there.'" This boundlessness can present other difficulties. People with dementia often become dizzy and disoriented. This may render some comfortable places awful and some strange places attractive. For the person with dementia, the world is filled with objects that appear as recalcitrant: the sock resists conformity with the foot, and the bracelet stubbornly refuses to fit over her hand. There are situations in which she is caught up in bodily intention, usually situations that call for dexterous

action. The researchers give the example of a person whose arms are held out for dancing and to which the person with dementia immediately responds.

Example 2: MS and Lived Space

The philosopher Kay Toombs (2001b), who suffers from multiple sclerosis (MS) herself, describes how, for her, body physical space is oriented space. Points in space do not represent merely objective positions, but rather they mark the varying range of her aims and gestures. The narrow passageway in which she has to move with her wheelchair represents a "restrictive potentiality" for her body requiring a modification of her actions. The dimensions of high and low also vary according to the position of her body. From her wheelchair, the top three shelves in the grocery store are too high to reach. To be a body is therefore to be tied to a certain world. Lived space thus concerns the encounter with an environing world: a world of places, things and situations that have meaning for living and consequently for health.

Linda Finlay describes the lifeworld of a woman in an attempt to elucidate the existential impact of early stage MS (Finlay 2003). She shows how the unity between her body and self can no longer be taken for granted. With her arm desensitized and spatially dislocated, she has to learn how to carry out everyday living tasks in new and unfamiliar ways. She must look at her arm in order to see what "it" is doing. This provokes a sense of bodily alienation. Also, she tries to keep her illness hidden from others; this part of her identity needs to be a secret and only emerges within her personal space when she is alone in bed at night.

Example 3: Lived Space in the Hospital

In my PhD study, I shadowed older patients during their stay in the hospital. Shadowing is an observational method in which the researcher observes an individual during a relatively long time. Central aspects of the method are the focus on meaning expressed by the whole body, and an extended stay of the researcher in the phenomenal event itself (van der Meide et al. 2013). I have described the essential structure of their experiences of hospitalization as "feeling an outsider left in uncertainty" (van der Meide et al. 2015). The use of the term "outsider" describes the feeling of "not fitting in" and "not belonging to." The hospital environment plays a constitutive role in this experience and appears as an inhospitable place. The opposite, a hospitable place, is a place where a person feels comfortable, involved in his or her own way and recognized as a person for whom the situation carries meaning.

Although the older patients experience the hospital as safe in certain respects, they do not feel at ease. The proximity of hospital staff provides reassurance that the physical state is being monitored and that help is at hand in case something goes wrong. However, the sense of safety seems strictly limited to their body in a physical sense. The observations show that hospital staff typically enter the room for a specific purpose: for example, to draw back the curtains in the morning, to take a blood pressure measurement or to shower the patient. Most of the conversations between care professionals and the older patient are functionally oriented. I witnessed many moments of self-talk in which the older patients were struggling aloud with their wishes and carefully evaluating them. Having the impression that care professionals are busy ("they continuously walk back and forth") seems to make the older patients reluctant to express their needs. They don't want to be a burden for the nurse. Diffidence about using the hospital button is an example of this ambiguous safety. On the one hand, the older patients know it can be used when nobody is around and help is needed, and on the other hand, they are uncertain about what they should use the bell for. Despite being constantly surrounded by many care professionals, the older patients feel alone when it comes to figuring out how to deal with the situation and much of their concerns and uncertainties remain unexpressed, although they would prefer it otherwise.

Consideration

What the foregoing shows is that space is not merely experienced from within, but that it has a profound impact on practices in the hospital and daily life by determining actions and behaviours. That is due to a number of features of space. Firstly, space *shapes and alters identities*. The meaning of MS is partly constituted by the space in which a person with MS moves. Also, space may *include and exclude*. Some people may feel comfortable and at ease in a given space, while others feel lost and alienated. This is eloquently described in the first example of the person with Alzheimer. Finally, space *creates possibilities and imposes restrictions*. Literal space configures possibilities for movement and action, as we have seen in the example of Toombs. If one is impaired and wheelchair bound, only surfaces that are accessible are conducive to this conveyance. The experiences of the older patients show that lived space is also related to autonomy and that it has relational meanings. The hospital appears as a closed space for older patients, rather than an open space that invites activity and involvement. The patients' worlds are thus not only objectively smaller as they are confined to the hospital bed or a chair but also subjectively contracted.

Space as an Active and Social Process

Care as a Practice

Care ethics has stressed the centrality of caring for human life as a practice. Within care ethics, care is not seen as an isolated act or a set of actions that just occurs between the patient and the healthcare professional. Indeed, care is not given in a societal vacuum. Society as such and politics in particular bring intentions and expectations to the matter of care giving, its institutions and its funding (Vosman and Baart, 2011). Since caring always involves power, it is political at every level (Tronto 2010). All kinds of other institutional incentives, such as market-orientation, accountability, cost-reduction and technologization, play an increasing role in the hospital, and consequently have implications for the healthcare professional-patient relationship (Vosman and Baart 2008).

As sociologist Andrew Sayer has noted, the dominant logic of systemic rationality changes the basis of our institutions. "Many of us are all too familiar with the rise of audits and the imposition of standardized procedures on activities which seem to defy standardization. Supposedly, these provide rational systems for organizing and assessing the performance of individuals and institutions" (Sayer 2011). Consequently, care can be understood as a practice that takes place in a complicated interplay of people, actions, artefacts (taken for granted) modes of knowledge and organizational structures (beyond the hospital as institution). A practice perspective implies that an issue can only be solved to some extent if one takes a sufficiently large perspective (a cut-out) and simultaneously addresses the question at different levels (Baart and Vosman 2015). The cultural anthropologists Gibson and Olarte Sierra show that hospital beds can be understood as spaces that are constituted through meaning and practice as political, socio-economical, cultural and social. The hospital bed might appear as an administrative space, a space of discipline and medical surveillance, but also of self-surveillance (Gibson and Olarte Sierra 2006).

Empirical studies performed from a lifeworld approach are predominantly focusing on the patient perspective. They state that descriptions offered by a lifeworld perspective revealing the experiences of those in need of care can make a difference to the deepening of emphatic understanding in readers and practitioners (Galvin and Todres 2013). The lifeworld perspective approaches care as an interaction between two people: the patient and the healthcare professional. The conceptualization of lifeworld-led healthcare includes an articulation of three dimensions: a philosophy of the person, a view of well-being and not just illness and a philosophy of care that is consistent with this. What is missing is a contextual and political dimension. Karin Dahlberg has emphasized that phenomenology is not studying the individual, but is studying how a particular phenomenon manifests and appears in the lifeworld, and this always already includes the social world (Dahlberg 2006). However, many phenomenological researchers tend to isolate the phenomenon under study from the context it is lived in by focusing too narrowly on individual experiences. This applies in particular to psychologically oriented phenomenological research. The social and political context usually plays an important role at the beginning of the research, in providing a rationale for conducting the study, and at the end, when the results are reflected upon. But throughout the whole research process, such as when choosing a particular method, while collecting the data and in the analysis, the context often receives little attention, as the focus remains on the individual experience.

Space as a Social Product

Henri Lefebvre (1901–1991) was a French philosopher and sociologist engaged with existential ideas (Elden 2004). In his prolific career, Lefebvre wrote more than 60 books and 300 articles covering a wide range of topics. In his work, Lefebvre shows an interest in the dialectic and he tends to work with three terms rather than the dualism of the two. He conceives the three as affecting each other simultaneously, without prioritizing one term over another. Instead of searching for a transcendence, a synthesis or a negation, he studies the continual movement between them. Lefebvre has written about space in *The Production of Space* (1974/1991). In this book, he argues that space is a social product, or a complex social construct (based on values and the social production of meanings), that affects spatial practices and perceptions. "(Social) space is a (social) product [...]; the space thus produced also serves as a tool of thought and of action [...] In addition to being a means of production it is also a means of control, and hence of domination, of power."

Although his work is complex and not about care practices, some of his insights might be helpful to better understand the meaning of space for humanizing healthcare. Lefebvre criticizes the binary notion of objective and lived space for still starting from the subjectivity of the ego. Lefebvre aims to a materialist version of phenomenology in which the epistemological perspective shifts from the subject that thinks, acts and experiences to the process of social production of thought, action and experience. According to him, space is fundamentally bound up with social reality. Space does not exist "in itself"; it is produced. Lefebvre proceeds from a relational concept of space and views space as a social product. This calls for an analysis that would include the social constellations, power relations and conflicts relevant in each situation. This would also imply the shift of the research perspective from space to processes of its production; the embrace of the multiplicity of spaces that are socially produced and made productive in social practices; and the focus on the contradictory, conflictual and, ultimately, political character of the processes of production of space.

How is (social) space then produced? Key to Lefebvre's theory is the view that the production of space can be divided into three dialectically interconnected dimensions: the perceived (perçu), the conceived (conçu) and the lived (vécu). All three concepts denote active and at once individual and social processes.

> Human beings do not stand before, or amidst, social space; they do not relate to the space of society as they might to a picture, a show, or a mirror. They know that they *have* a space and that they *are* in this space. They do not merely enjoy a vision, a contemplation, a spectacle – for they act and situate themselves in space as active participants. (Lefebvre 1991, p. 294)

The first dimension is the perceived. Evidently, perception depends upon the subject: a patient does not experience the hospital in the same way as a medical doctor. Nevertheless, Lefebvre's attitude towards the phenomenological version of perception is quite sceptical. Therefore, he combines it with the concept of spatial practice in order to show that perception not only takes place in the mind, but that it is based on a concrete, produced materiality. The complex spatial organization of practices shapes perceived spaces in, for example, households, neighbourhoods and in hospitals. This is the physical dimension of space. Second, space cannot be perceived as such without having been conceived in thought previously. It refers to our knowledge of a certain space that is primarily produced by discourses of power and ideology constructed by professionals, researchers, policymakers etc. Space presumes an act of thought that is linked to the production of knowledge. This is the mental dimension of space. The dimension of lived space denotes the world as it is experienced by human beings in the practice of their everyday life. On this point, Lefebvre is unequivocal: the lived, practical experience cannot itself be exhausted through theoretical analysis. There always remains a surplus, a remainder.

Lefebvre's theory of the production of space identifies three moments of production: first, material production; second, the production of knowledge; and third, the production of meaning. Space is to be understood in an active sense as an intricate web of relationships that is continuously produced and reproduced. When we approach space as something that is produced, rather than just something that is experienced by individuals, the object of the analysis should consequently be the active process of production.

Conclusion

What can be gained from such a three-dimensional perspective of space when studying the (de)humanization of hospital care? The Norwegian philosopher Kari Martinsen (2006) has described the hospital as a public house that expresses a common order. This order expresses in its turn that which has been valued in society. She speaks about the battle for the spaces and the tension between the rooms of the hospital as spaces in which to dwell and spaces in which to be disciplined. Dwelling refers to the feeling of belonging and being safe, and it concerns a shared space, while a disciplined space refers to a means of control and domination. In this context, she distinguishes two ways of seeing by the healthcare professional, which she calls the perceiving eye and the recording eye. Perceiving should be seen as a participating way of looking at the other and allows the other, who is often not known, to emerge. Perception is a fundamental openness towards the other, and it is the patient who has the initiative to show what is of importance. In perceiving, there is a unity between the one who perceives and that which is perceived, and it puts the healthcare professional and the patient in a common world. It thus goes deeper than having good communication skills and requires an open attitude on the part of the healthcare professional. Indeed, a good healthcare professional should not only hear what is explicitly asked for but should be sensitive to implicit appeals (Vosman and Baart 2011).

The second way of seeing Martinsen describes is recording. While perceiving occurs within a relation, recording takes place from an outside position. The "eye" of the healthcare professional is then busy with looking for and abstracting common characteristics to organize under an already defined concept of classification. It abstracts from the concrete context. The origin of the verb "to diagnose" refers to this analytical scrutiny that abstracts from all the details that might obscure a clear view (van Heijst 2011). Diagnosis means looking *through* something instead of looking *at* someone. This leads to a specific understanding of the situation. Evidently, many diagnostic tools and screening instruments have greatly contributed to the progress that medicine has achieved since the seventeenth century. However, we should not ignore some of the consequences of this view, of which one is the nature of space that is produced by such an approach. Over-emphasis on diagnostics and guidelines guides the physical and the mental dimension of space in a certain direction, following the dominant ideology of society and politics. Also, the logic of the market, for example, requires that doctors do not spend any time with the patient that is not being paid for.

An increased interest in the dimension of space in care can be observed. The dominant objective of contemporary hospital architecture is to create a "pleasant and sustaining environment." Hospitals do everything possible to resemble a hospital as little as possible. One may notice this already when one enters the hospital. Although the hospital has always been a public space, this has acquired another connotation in recent years. The ground floor of hospitals increasingly looks like an extension of the city centre, with interior streets and commercial facilities, ATMs, bars and hairdressers. This has been called the "malling" of the hospital (Fiset 2006). Healing architecture draws upon research that shows that environmental elements such as natural light, a view of nature, less noise and subdued colours produce positive patient outcomes and reduce stress. Single-patient rooms not only create a quieter hospital stay and increase privacy but also reduce patient transfers and the risk of infection. A family zone where family members may stay overnight helps patients feel less alone. A quieter environment may also help staff perform their duties with fewer medical errors. In order to determine whether these developments are good examples of humanized care, a thorough analysis is needed. The three-dimensional perspective of space, as described in this paper, may provide a guide for such an analysis and can illuminate care as a practice that is always social and political, but at the same time lived out in the lifeworld. It offers a lens to look at, reflect on and enhance care practices. Also, studying the dynamic interplay between the dimensions enables a better understanding of spatial vulnerability.

References

Alzhén, R. (2011). Illness as Unhomelike Being-in-the-World. Phenomenology and Medical Practice. *Medicine, Health Care, and Philosophy, 14*(3), 323–331.

Ashworth, A., & Ashworth, P. (2003). The Lifeworld as Phenomenon and as Research Heuristic, Exemplified by a Study of the Lifeworld of a Person Suffering Alzheimer's Disease. *Journal of Phenomenological Psychology, 34*(2), 179–204.

Baart, A., & Vosman, F. (Eds.). (2015). *De Patient Terug van Weggeweest. Werken Aan Menslievende Zorg in Het Ziekenhuis*. Amsterdam: SWP.

Berglund, M., Westin, L., Svanström, R., & Sundler, A. J. (2012). Suffering Caused by Care—Patients' Experiences from Hospital Settings. *International Journal of Qualitative Studies on Health and Well-Being, 7*, 1–9.

Cassell, E. J. (2001). The Phenomenon of Suffering and Its Relationship to Pain. In S. K. Toombs (Ed.), *Handbook of Phenomenology and Medicine* (pp. 371–390). Dordrecht: Kluwer Academic Publishers.

Dahlberg, K. (2006). The Individual in the World—The World in the Individual: Towards a Human Science Phenomenology that Includes the Social World. *Indo-Pacific Journal of Phenomenology, 6*, 1–9.

Dahlberg, K., Todres, L., & Galvin, K. (2009). Lifeworld-Led Healthcare Is More Than Patient-Led Care: An Existential View of Well-Being. *Medicine, Health Care, and Philosophy, 12*(3), 265–271.

Elden, S. (2004). *Understanding Henri Lefebvre*. London: Continuum.

Finlay, L. (2003). The Intertwining of Body, Self and World: A Phenomenological Study of Living with Recently-Diagnosed Multiple Sclerosis. *Journal of Phenomenological Psychology, 34*(2), 157–178.

Finlay, L. (2011). *Phenomenology for Therapists: Researching the Lived World*. Oxford: Wiley-Blackwell.

Fiset, M. (2006). Hospitabel Hospitals: Creating a Healing Environment. International Hospital Federation Reference Book. Retrieved from http://www.fisethospiconsult.com/SCN_0002.pdf

Galvin, K., & Todres, L. (2013). *Caring and Well-Being. A Lifeworld Approach*. New York: Routledge.

Gibson, D., & Olarte Sierra, M. F. (2006). The Hospital Bed as Space. Observations from South Africa and the Netherlands. *Medische Antropologie, 18*(1), 161–176.

Hansen, F. (2015). The Philosophical Practitioner as Co-researcher. In A. Fatic & L. Amir (Eds.), *Practicing Philosophy* (pp. 22–41). Newcastle: Cambridge Scholars Publishing.

Heidegger, M. (1998). *Zijn En Tijd (Being and Time)* (M. Wildschut, Trans.). Nijmegen: SUN.
Husserl, E. (1970). *The Crisis of European Sciences and Transcendental Phenomenology. An Introduction to Phenomenological Philosophy*. Evanston: Northwestern University Press.
Lefebvre, H. (1991). *The Production of Space*. Oxford: Blackwell.
Martinsen, K. (2006). *Care and Vulnerability*. Oslo: Akribe.
Merleau-Ponty, M. (1962). *Phenomenology of Perception*. Abingdon: Routledge.
Norlyk, A., Martinsen, B., & Dahlberg, K. (2013). Getting to Know Patients' Lived Space. *Indo-Pacific Journal of Phenomenology, 13*(2), 1–12.
Sayer, A. (2011). *Why Things Matter to People. Social Science, Values and Ethical Life*. Cambridge: Cambridge University Press.
Sokolowski, R. (2000). *Introduction to Phenomenology*. Cambridge: Cambridge University Press.
Svenaeus, F. (2000). The Body Uncanny—Further Steps Towards a Phenomenology of Illness. *Medicine, Health Care, and Philosophy, 3*(2), 125–137.
Svenaeus, F. (2011). Illness as Unhomelike-Being-in-the-World: Heidegger and the Phenomenology of Medicine. *Medicine, Health Care, and Philosophy, 14*(3), 333–343.
Todres, L., Galvin, K. T., & Dahlberg, K. (2007). Lifeworld-Led Healthcare: Revisiting a Humanizing Philosophy that Integrates Emerging Trends. *Medicine, Health Care, and Philosophy, 10*(1), 53–63.
Todres, L., Galvin, K. T., & Holloway, I. (2009). The Humanization of Healthcare: A Value Framework for Qualitative Research. *International Journal of Qualitative Studies on Health and Well-Being, 4*(2), 68–77.
Toombs, S. K. (Ed.). (2001a). *Handbook of Phenomenology and Medicine*. Dordrecht: Kluwer Academic Publishers.
Toombs, S. K. (2001b). Reflections on Bodily Change: The Lived Experience of Disability. In S. K. Toomb (Ed.), *Handbook of Phenomenology and Medicine* (pp. 247–262). Dordrecht: Kluwer Academic Publishers.
Tronto, J. C. (2010). Creating Caring Institutions: Politics, Plurality, and Purpose. *Ethics and Social Welfare, 4*(2), 158–171.
Van der Meide, H., Leget, C., & Olthuis, G. (2013). Giving Voice to Vulnerable People: The Value of Shadowing for Phenomenological Healthcare Research. *Medicine, Health Care, and Philosophy, 16*(4), 731–737.
Van der Meide, H., Olthuis, G., & Leget, C. (2015). Feeling an Outsider Left in Uncertainty—A Phenomenological Study on the Experiences of Older Hospital Patients. *Scandinavian Journal of Caring Sciences, 29*(3), 528–536.

Van Heijst, A. (2011). *Professional Loving Care. An Ethical View of the Healthcare Sector*. Leuven: Peeters.

Van Manen, M. (2014). *Phenomenology of Practice*. Walnut Creek: Left Coast Press.

Verghese, A. (2011). A Doctor's Touch. *TED Talk*. Retrieved June 1, 2016, from https://www.ted.com/talks/abraham_verghese_a_doctor_s_touch. Published 2011.

Visse, M. (2012). *Openings for Humanization in Modern Health Care Practices*. Unpublished dissertation. Amsterdam: Vrije Universiteit. https://research.vu.nl/ws/portalfiles/portal/682632.

Vosman, F., & Baart, A. (2008). *Aannemelijke Zorg Over Het Uitzieden En Verdringen van Praktische Wijsheid in de Gezondheidszorg*. Den Haag: Lemma.

Vosman, F., & Baart, A. (2011). Relationship Based Care and Recognition. Part Two: Good Care and Recognition. In C. Leget, C. Gastmans, & M. Verkerk (Eds.), *Care, Compassion and Recognition: An Ethical Dimension* (pp. 201–228). Leuven: Peeters.

Williams, A. N., & Irurita, V. (2004). Therapeutic and Non-therapeutic Interpersonal Interactions: The Patient's Perspective. *Journal of Clinical Nursing, 13*(7), 806–815.

Open Access This book is licensed under the terms of the Creative Commons Attribution 4.0 International License (http://creativecommons.org/licenses/by/4.0/), which permits use, sharing, adaptation, distribution and reproduction in any medium or format, as long as you give appropriate credit to the original author(s) and the source, provide a link to the Creative Commons license and indicate if changes were made.

The images or other third party material in this chapter are included in the chapter's Creative Commons license, unless indicated otherwise in a credit line to the material. If material is not included in the chapter's Creative Commons license and your intended use is not permitted by statutory regulation or exceeds the permitted use, you will need to obtain permission directly from the copyright holder.

Conclusion: Asking the Right Questions

Joachim Boldt, Annelieke Driessen, Björn Freter, Tobias Haeusermann, Franziska Krause, Pei-Yi Liu, Tim Opgenhaffen, and Annekatrin Skeide

Care is an important part of daily healthcare practices and the self-understanding of those working in the healthcare sector. At the same time, the notion of care carries an extraordinary range of distinctive meanings, as the preceding chapters have made clear. Indeed, definitions of care and its associated practices have often been so broad that

---

This conclusion was jointly written by the following contributors to this book (in alphabetical order): Boldt, Joachim; Driessen, Annelieke; Freter, Björn; Haeusermann, Tobias; Krause, Franziska; Liu, Pei-Yi; Opgenhaffen, Tim; Skeide, Annekatrin. Tobias deserves special mention for writing the first draft.

J. Boldt (✉) • F. Krause
Department of Medical Ethics and the History of Medicine, University of Freiburg, Freiburg, Germany

A. Driessen
Amsterdam Institute for Social Science Research (AISSR), University of Amsterdam, Amsterdam, The Netherlands

B. Freter
Independent Scholar, Berlin, Germany

© The Author(s) 2018
F. Krause, J. Boldt (eds.), *Care in Healthcare*,
https://doi.org/10.1007/978-3-319-61291-1_14

care may be found everywhere and in everything, including at times in the most unexpected places. Alternately, definitions have also been so narrow that one finds it hard to go beyond a limited set of questions, remaining instead within the confines of a single discipline. Although this makes it difficult to come up with a precise definition of care, it does not imply that it is impossible to describe care in words at all.

The philosophical and ethical accounts in part one of this book agree that the dyadic relation between a person in need and a person who provides help is one of the core elements of care. For example, in her contribution, Krause demonstrates how the account of interpersonal relationality supplied by the philosopher and phenomenologist Emmanuel Levinas can be useful for discussions of care in healthcare ethics. Levinas claims that any encounter with another person inherently involves having to assume responsibilities for this other person. In the same vein, by drawing on the conceptual resources of phenomenology, Freter lays bare basic structures of the encounter of one person with another in his analysis of the biblical story of the Good Samaritan. The hermeneutic tradition often stresses that the way in which humans epistemically and physically relate to one another is reciprocal and invokes relational dependencies, with the writings of Paul Ricoeur serving as a prime example of this. In his analysis, Boldt describes and interprets these relational dependencies within Ricoeur's concept of the self. In his chapter, Maio shows how Ricoeur's approach is closely connected to the detailed understandings of

---

T. Haeusermann
Epidemiology, Biostatistics & Prevention Institute (EBPI), University of Zürich, Zürich, Switzerland

P.-Y. Liu
Faculty of Nursing, Philosophisch-Theologische Hochschule Vallendar (PTHV), Vallendar, Germany

T. Opgenhaffen
Institute for Social Law, Katholieke Universiteit Leuven, Leuven, Belgium

A. Skeide
Human and Health Sciences, University of Bremen, Bremen, Germany

care that Joan Tronto develops in her political theory of care. Finally, in her reconstruction of historical precursors to today's thinking in care ethics, Conradi unveils the significant contributions of reflections about care made by Jewish women who were part of the social care and social reform movements of the late nineteenth and early twentieth century. As Conradi argues, these often overlooked reflections are closely connected, for example, to the theory of the I-You-relation as devised by the Jewish philosopher and theologian Martin Buber.

Even if one assumes that it is possible to point to core elements of care, as the chapters in part one of the book attempt to do, these descriptions alone cannot supply simple solutions to the challenges that are rooted in the ambivalences and tensions of the notion of care in healthcare. Sociologists and anthropologists, among others, have long been interested in showing how extensive, situated, and complex care can be. The chapters in part two of this book address questions that arise in these disciplines, as well as in disciplines such as nursing sciences and law, including: If there is a situation in which a caregiver reacts to another person's needs and provides help, can the care practices include coercion? And if so, when and where is this the case? Is care compatible with exclusion? Can it be passive or invisible? Can it be incorporated into standardised and regulated routines? Can the care vocabulary be adapted to medical terminology?

Looking back at all of the chapters in this book, the following key ambivalences and tensions of care in healthcare emerge:

Caring, Influencing, and Coercing

Caring for another person necessarily implies influencing the other person's abilities or their desires. For example, someone who receives help may be able to do what they could not do before. He or she might be in a better mood, experience gratitude, or feel burdened by social expectations to repay the help that was received. When the caregiver and care receiver discuss rehabilitative or therapeutic options, they imagine and perhaps adjust what they want for themselves and for one another accordingly.

Sometimes the actions that a caregiver considers to be in the overall interest of the care receiver might not coincide with the initial will of the person receiving care. Nobody doubts that a nurse who supports the daily activities of someone who is temporarily or permanently disabled is providing care. Care is self-evident here. It is the nurse's job. But what if the nurse tricks a patient who does not want to get up into getting up anyway? Although providing care in this case may appear paternalistic, can it still be a response to a need? As Driessen's chapter exemplifies, in these cases, caregiving may include attempts to influence a patient's wishes, to encourage him or her not only to stop resisting what the caregiver perceives to be good care, but to actually want it. The line that separates these practices from practices involving unjustified manipulation or even coercion is a fine one. Indeed, Driessen contends that with regard to dementia, good care involves attempting to avoid coercion, even if such attempts sometimes fail.

Writing about the psychiatric emergency ward, Opgenhaffen argues that is not always self-evident that coercion never can be part of good care. In search of an ethical foundation for handling coercion, he maintains that in extreme cases, coercion which aims at restoring autonomy might, in fact, be conducted in a caring way. Although from a care perspective manipulation and coercion must, prima facie, be avoided, since they harm another person both physically and psychologically, even these actions may be justifiable from the point of view of care if there is immediate danger to the life and health of others or of the person concerned. As Opgenhaffen points out, clearly identifying and defining such circumstances, and maintaining a caring attitude that places the needs of the person in question before safety concerns, may help to minimise the dehumanising aspects of coercion.

Drawing the line between justifiably influencing the will of a care receiver in order to maintain what one regards to be the person's overall well-being on the one hand, and manipulation and coercion on the other hand, is tantamount to making a distinction between the kinds of relationality that are constitutive of, or at least compatible with, human autonomy and the kinds of relationality that impede autonomy. As Boldt argues, autonomy is based on social conditions and comprises elements of social dependencies. It is therefore a mistake to place valuing autonomy in opposition to valuing care. If one is concerned about the autonomy of oneself and others, one ought to be concerned as well about the well-being of oneself and others, and the care provided to oneself and others. Still, it is impossible to define this approach in abstract terms. Instead continuous everyday reflective and practical efforts are needed when providing care in healthcare settings.

Care, Inclusion, and Exclusion

At first glance, care practices seem to be prime examples of inclusive activities. When caring for another person, one turns to another person, appreciates their needs and interests, and acts in an attempt to improve their situation. Such acts ideally enable care receivers to keep up their daily lives and thus to maintain or return to their positions as members of all those social groups to which they belong.

Nonetheless, care may also contribute to social exclusion. As the dementia village described by Haeusermann exemplifies, care receivers may feel happy in surroundings that in effect exclude them from their own neighbourhoods and social groups. Haeusermann points out that while the dementia village aims to give its inhabitants the impression of an inclusive, "normal" village life, this village is also surrounded by a fence.

Is it appropriate to isolate certain vulnerable groups from the majority at a societal level? When approaching this question, it soon becomes clear that a one-dimensional conception of social exclusion does not lead to fruitful results. Rather, we need to consider the multiple levels at which exclusion and inclusion are realised simultaneously. People with dementia can be included by virtue of a state's provision of affordable medical care. At the same time, they can be excluded from their local community or family through a gated institution. Meanwhile, the elderly can remain included in their social network by living with their families or within community care projects, but be denied appropriate medical care offered by the state. Future analyses of care and care practices need to take a close look at exclusion that stems from caring, its relation to the individual will, and its effects on individual well-being and on societal cohesion.

Care, Passivity, and Invisibility

Is what we call care always visible? Sometimes it is visible in what is done. In those cases passivity may appear to indicate a neglect of care. However, upon closer inspection, passivity can be a very important part of care as well. The most obvious example is listening to and observing what a patient says or expresses nonverbally. Care always involves phases of passivity in which one gets to know the other person and his or her preferences and needs. What is more, in some cases, passively being with, observing, and not intervening can be considered an integral part of actively caring, as Skeide demonstrates in her contribution on midwifes who accompany labouring women. Here, being with can be understood as a caring intervention.

In other cases, it might be helpful if care receivers are not aware of the caregiver's presence. Care in these cases is supplied by making itself invisible. The policy in the dementia care village described by Haeusermann prescribed that care workers work without uniforms. In the dementia village, what is allowed to be visible is the "normal", common structure of typical everyday life in the German countryside (or at least the stereotypical, utopian conception of it). Meant to support the inhabitants' well-being, this nonetheless resulted in uneasiness among some care workers, who felt the policy nullified their educational efforts. Moreover, for the residents and their family members, the absence of a clear care authority could lead to situations in which they do not know who to turn to.

In general terms, although care might at times appear to be invisible or passive, only the person who is seeking care can determine whether such invisible or passive care constitutes neglect or reassurance. The ambivalence between caring actively and passively, visibly and invisibly, thus requires a cautious approach in any analysis of instances in which care is provided.

Care, Regulation, Standardisation, and Fragmentation

Care in healthcare is a professional activity that takes place in a context of regulation and standardisation. This helps to safeguard, among other things, patient rights, a just distribution of care provisions, and the long-term economic stability of the healthcare system. Nonetheless, regulation can interfere with the provision of optimal care in individual cases. Moreover, following regulations without understanding their relation to the value of care can lead to attitudes and actions that neglect this value. As mentioned above with regard to coercion in psychiatry, Opgenhaffen contends that if coercion is understood as a borderline case of care in which one still needs to take into account the well-being of the patient, this can help to minimise the dehumanising aspects of coercive measures.

What is more, given the importance of the individual and personal aspects of giving and receiving care, it will always be necessary to balance abstract regulation on the one hand and individual context-sensitive decisions on the other hand. This is to say that regulating care in healthcare settings must always leave room for responsible, individual decisions by the caregiver.

Standardised care practices often go hand in hand with fragmented distributions of responsibility and authority. As Liu shows with respect to ambulant diabetes care, nurses are responsible for the daily care and well-being of their patients in many respects. At the same time, their authority to administer therapies is limited, and patients accordingly do not regard nursing staff recommendations as authoritative expert statements on par with the statements of physicians.

Finally, standardisation does not only have an effect on the relation of caregiver to care receiver. As van der Meide argues, it also concerns the spaces in which care is provided. Although rooms and routines in the hospital are needed to facilitate efficient care procedures, standardised spaces may also compromise the well-being and healing processes of patients.

Care, Language, and Ambiguity

Communication in healthcare is dominated by medical terminology, which aims to precisely define and refer to diseases, therapies, and physiological facts. This terminology and its aims are an indispensable part of statistical surveys, economic classifications as well as efficient and error-free expert communication. In contrast, the language that is used to denote practices of care and the language that is used in providing care can appear to lack this kind of precision.

Since care practices are part of an institutional setting that involves experts, distribution of labour, and expert exchanges, some would argue that a lack of precision represents a disadvantage. In this context, they would surmise that care language needs to strive for accuracy just as medical terminology does. At the same time, however, the language of care that is used in care practices is necessarily close to everyday language since it has to do with everyday activities that are not confined to the healthcare setting. Moreover, it involves the experiences and perceptions of patients as described in their own words. The way patients express their experiences can vary according to their prior life experiences, their convictions, and their knowledge. The vocabulary they use may be part of a larger narrative, rather than comprising single terms that refer to clearly delineable states of affairs. As the relevant discourses show, the value of narrative self-identity, embodied knowledge, and patient knowledge should not be neglected.

While this ultimately may be an unresolvable tension, Kohlen highlights the fact that in today's healthcare settings, striving for accuracy prevails over the acceptance of ambiguity. Given the focus on economic measures, core elements of care that are subject to ambiguity are often regarded as irrelevant. The voices of caregivers are thus underrepresented in todays' healthcare institutions, as Kohlen demonstrates in the case of hospital ethics committees.

Concluding Remarks

Identifying and describing the tensions and ambivalences of care, as this book has done, is not tantamount to resolving these issues. Indeed, as has been argued, many of the tensions described may be inevitable and unresolvable both in theory and in practice. Anyone working in and thinking about today's healthcare settings will always be challenged in their self-understanding and daily practices to find ways to adequately deal with these tensions. However, asking the right questions may open doors to more attuned understandings of the complexities and challenges of care. To pose these questions and deal with these challenges, then, is a form of caring about care. This is what this book aimed to do.

Open Access This chapter is licensed under the terms of the Creative Commons Attribution 4.0 International License (http://creativecommons.org/licenses/by/4.0/), which permits use, sharing, adaptation, distribution and reproduction in any medium or format, as long as you give appropriate credit to the original author(s) and the source, provide a link to the Creative Commons license and indicate if changes were made.

The images or other third party material in this chapter are included in the chapter's Creative Commons license, unless indicated otherwise in a credit line to the material. If material is not included in the chapter's Creative Commons license and your intended use is not permitted by statutory regulation or exceeds the permitted use, you will need to obtain permission directly from the copyright holder.

Index

A

accountability, 273
alienation, 99, 172–4, 196, 198, 200, 203, 271
Alzheimer's disease, 111, 135, 159n10, 270, 271, 273
ambiguity, 58–60, 176, 194, 195, 267, 269, 290
ambivalences, 5, 7, 8, 58, 137, 224, 285, 288, 290
anger, 198, 227, 241
appeals, 6, 37–45, 53, 69, 123–5, 181, 183, 196, 277
attentiveness, 4, 13, 14, 28n2, 46n6, 52, 58, 61, 78, 81, 82, 94, 98, 101, 102, 116–18, 120–2, 125, 127, 136, 147, 148, 150, 170, 174, 179, 192, 213, 222, 239, 243, 244, 246, 258, 270, 275
attitudes, 4, 28n3, 44, 52, 53, 58, 60, 78, 79, 81, 84, 91, 93, 94, 98, 117, 129n12, 155, 183, 250, 267, 276, 277, 286, 289
authorities, 7, 17, 140, 155, 172, 213–15, 218–20, 225, 226, 230, 239, 243, 246, 288, 289
autonomy, 6, 7, 65–9, 81, 83, 84, 90, 97, 98, 161n17, 162n21, 173, 182–4, 216, 221, 230, 256, 273, 286, 287
awareness, 53, 55, 62, 94, 112, 151, 213, 220, 224, 229, 230, 266

B

Beauchamp, T.L., 66, 79, 97
beneficence, 79
bodily interaction, 202

Note: Page number followed by 'n' denote notes.

© The Author(s) 2018
F. Krause, J. Boldt (eds.), *Care in Healthcare*,
https://doi.org/10.1007/978-3-319-61291-1

body, 4, 44, 67, 92, 93, 99, 100, 114, 117, 124, 125, 137, 148, 160n12, 161n20, 171, 191, 192, 194, 196–8, 200, 201, 204, 205, 205n1, 213, 244, 257, 259, 266–9, 271, 272
Buber, M., 14–19, 28n3, 285

C

care, 1–8, 13–27, 37–45, 51–62, 65, 87–103, 112, 136, 137, 150, 157, 159n8, 161n21, 169, 191, 211, 237–51, 265
care-givers, 40, 42–5, 47n9, 239, 244
care practices, 5, 7, 94, 116, 125, 128n6, 129n9, 137, 160n12, 211, 238, 245, 266, 268, 275, 278, 285, 287–90
care receivers, 1, 2, 4, 5, 7, 53, 94, 117, 215, 220–2, 231n5, 244, 286–9
care relation, 53, 124, 215, 216, 225
care situations, 4, 127, 213, 218, 224, 227
care workers, 111–13, 116–18, 120, 122, 123, 125, 126, 128n6, 129n9, 129n11, 129n12, 130n19, 130n20, 131n22, 159n8, 288
Cassell, E.J., 266
Childress, J.F., 66, 79
coercion, 113, 116, 118, 125, 126, 129n12, 173, 177, 285, 286, 289
Cohen, H., 14, 16–19, 28n4
commodification, 89, 103n3, 221
compassion, 14, 39, 46n2
competences, 52, 59, 94, 155, 170, 180, 194, 200, 206n6, 224, 228, 241, 257
concerns, 18, 37–45, 55, 68, 84, 90, 138, 143, 153, 156, 181, 222–4, 238–47, 253–7, 259, 268, 271, 272, 277, 286, 289
Conradi, E., 2, 6, 13, 52, 285
consents, 66, 67, 89, 129n9, 171
consumers, 212, 220, 222, 232n8
customers, 206n7, 213, 215, 220, 223, 229, 230, 231n5

D

decision-making, 71, 73, 74, 76, 77, 82, 83, 85, 113–15, 205, 230n1, 240, 246, 247
dependency, 55, 56, 62, 92, 93, 117, 173, 196, 285, 287
Derrida, J., 104n7, 193
diabetes, 43, 44, 211–30, 289
diseases, 5, 44, 79, 80, 135, 147, 212, 215, 216, 221, 223, 230, 240, 244, 245, 258, 266, 290
Durkheim, E., 156

E

efficiency, 151, 213, 224, 229
embodied, 191, 244, 290
embodiment, 88, 205n1, 268
empathy, 13, 256
empowering, 212, 221, 252
equality, 19, 53, 55, 101, 102, 170, 180

ethics, 2, 6–8, 13, 46n5, 51, 65, 66, 69–71, 73, 74, 77, 80, 83, 85n3, 87–91, 102, 103, 117, 162n21, 169, 211, 237–9, 248, 250, 258, 273, 284, 285
ethnography, 115, 117, 136, 137, 154, 159n11, 163n25, 195, 212, 239
exclusion, 7, 151, 158n1, 287, 288

F

Fabre, C., 89, 90
Foucault, M., 159
fragmentation, 175, 183, 241–3, 269, 289
freedom, 7, 68, 72, 73, 90, 93, 95, 113, 138, 143, 156, 170, 173, 180, 213
frustration, 220, 227, 241

G

Gallagher, A., 237
Gemeinschaft (community), 137, 151–7
Gesellschaft (society), 137, 151
Gilligan, C., 46n5, 51, 52, 55, 60, 117, 173, 237

H

Hamelin, Germany, 136–9, 160n14
Heidegger, M., 104n6, 266, 267, 269
Hochschild, A.R., 88, 100, 117, 130n17
home-based care, 211
hospitals, 2, 8, 136, 171, 172, 174, 176, 177, 179, 195, 198, 203–5, 212, 215, 237–51, 265, 266, 270, 276–8, 289
hospital environment, 8, 272
hospital ethics committee (HEC), 8, 237–51, 290
hospitality, 13, 97
humanization of care, 265–78
Husserl, E., 267, 268

I

inclusion, 7, 151, 237, 287, 288
indication, medical, 67
institution, 3, 7, 60, 76, 101, 102, 136, 151, 153, 170, 175, 182, 221, 239, 242, 244, 245, 247, 249, 251, 253, 273, 274, 287, 290
institutional hierarchy, 199, 213, 218, 225, 230, 230n1, 230n2, 256–8
institutional rules, 4
institutionalization, 4, 102, 243, 252
interdependency, 65–85, 103, 117, 170, 173, 183
invisibility, 4, 129n11, 181, 182, 204, 226, 239, 240, 245, 288

J

Jewish ethics, 6, 13–18
Jewish society, 23
Jewish women's league, 24, 26
Judaism, 16, 17, 19, 20

K

Kant, I., 57, 73–5, 92
Kohlen, H., 7, 46n2, 211, 237–51, 290

L

law, 16, 17, 74, 101, 114, 129n8, 175, 177, 178, 182, 285
Leder, D., 197
Lefebvre, H., 8, 266, 275, 276
Lévinas, E., 7, 53, 58, 91–103, 207n13, 284
liberty, 89, 90, 98
lived space, 266, 267, 275, 276

M

maleficence, 79
marginalization, 253
medical ethics, 65, 66, 79, 80, 91
Merleau-Ponty, M., 267
midwifery, 2, 7, 191
Mill, J.S., 67–9, 71–3, 83, 84
Mol, A., 5, 116, 118, 124, 212, 213, 221–4
moral distress, 224, 241–3
Morgenstern, L., 24

N

need, 3, 4, 6, 14, 15, 18, 39, 52–7, 74–6, 78, 80–2, 84, 93, 94, 100, 102, 138, 140, 143, 172, 179, 180, 212, 221, 239, 240, 247, 258, 271, 274, 288, 290
Noddings, N., 46n5, 159n7, 170, 172, 173, 176, 177, 180, 181, 237
normativity, 6, 37, 41
nurse, 7, 8, 38, 42, 45, 46n7, 47n8, 170, 175, 180, 211, 237–51, 272, 286, 289
nursing, 8, 27n1, 28n2, 37–45, 45n1, 46n7, 47n8, 47n10
nursing homes, 114, 116, 128n8, 136

P

Pappenheim, B., 24
Parkinson's disease, 135
participation, 8, 196, 199, 237, 238, 246–51, 254, 258
passivity, 95, 97, 205, 268, 288
patient's, 3–5, 8, 43, 44, 47n12, 56, 57, 61, 62, 65–8, 73, 78–80, 82–5, 123, 152, 163n25, 171–6, 178–80, 183, 211–24, 226–9, 230n1, 232n8, 239, 241–6, 249, 252, 254, 256–8, 265, 266, 268, 272–4, 277, 278, 286, 288–90
patient-physician relationship, 223
phenomenology, 37–45, 91, 92, 100, 267–73, 284
political engagement, 25
Pols, J., 116, 130n16, 163n25, 205
power, 60, 62, 77, 93, 117, 118, 126, 154, 199, 213, 225, 226, 229, 243, 257, 270, 273, 276
power relationships, 246, 250, 258
pregnancy, 87, 90, 91, 93, 99, 100, 104n8, 197, 198, 203, 204, 206n7, 208n18
principlism, 51, 55, 56, 59, 61, 62
professional care, 2, 128n5, 223, 225, 227, 230

psychiatry, 173, 289

Q

quality of care, 213, 222, 230n1, 232n8

R

recognition, 44, 55, 57, 96, 98, 100, 176, 229
regulations, 4, 7, 66, 67, 88, 103, 169–84, 229, 231n5, 289
relational autonomy, 96–8
residents, 7, 111–18, 120–3, 125, 126, 128n5, 128n6, 129n9, 129n12, 130n19, 131n22, 136–48, 150, 152, 153, 159n8, 159n10, 177, 161n16–n18
responsibility, 1, 7, 54, 62, 89, 92–6, 99, 100, 102, 170, 172, 179, 183, 199, 202, 214–16, 218, 223, 225–7, 230, 238, 240, 243, 247, 253, 256, 289
responsiveness, 58, 94, 170, 238
Ricoeur, P., 6, 52–4, 60, 62, 76, 81, 83, 85n4, 85n5, 285

S

Samaritan, 6, 39, 40
seclusion, 7, 169
self, 6, 53, 54, 76, 81, 92–101, 103, 104n6, 158n1, 179, 182, 183, 200, 201, 207n11, 207n13, 224, 266, 271
self-awareness, 54
self-sacrifice, 25
social reform, 6, 285
standardization, 4, 274, 289
surrogacy, 7, 87
Susman, M., 16
Svenaeus, F., 266

T

Talmud, 23
technologization, 273
tension, 112, 151, 152, 192, 215, 217, 219, 220, 222, 225, 227, 277, 290
Tönebön am See, Germany, 137
Toombs, S.K., 266, 271, 273
transcendence, 275
Tronto, J., 3, 46n2, 52, 79, 93, 94, 117, 170, 172, 173, 175, 179, 180, 182, 221, 229, 238, 245

U

utilitarianism, 92

V

Verkerk, M., 171, 173
virtue ethics, 51–2
Volition, 37–45
Vosman, F., 27n1, 273, 274, 277
vulnerability, 53, 92, 97, 99, 180, 240, 265, 269, 278

W

well-being, 2–8, 41, 43, 44, 66, 68, 74, 78–80, 82, 84, 85, 146, 174, 176, 180, 239, 253, 274, 286, 288, 289
will, 5, 7, 40, 42, 73, 74, 76, 78, 81, 83, 84, 111–27
will-formation, 72, 74, 75, 77, 81, 83, 84
witnessing, 7, 191–205

www.ingramcontent.com/pod-product-compliance
Lightning Source LLC
LaVergne TN
LVHW082118200926
848484LV00008B/1979